The Miracle of Natural Hormones
3rd Edition

Arthritis, Autoimmune Disorders, Chronic
Fatigue, Fibromyalgia, Heart Disease,
Hypothyroidism, Menopause, Anti-Aging
and Much More!

The Miracle of
Natural Hormones
3rd Edition

See How A Holistic Program Can:

- *Improve Your Energy*

- *Help You Overcome Chronic Illness*

- *Achieve Your Optimum Health*

David Brownstein, M.D.

With Over 50 Actual Case Studies!

For further copies of **The Miracle of Natural Hormones, 3rd Edition**:

Call: **1-888-647-5616** or send a check or money order in the amount of: $25.00 ($20.00 plus $5.00 shipping and handling) or for Michigan residents $26.20 ($20.00) plus $5.00 shipping and handling, plus $1.20 sales tax) to:

Medical Alternatives Press
4054 Oak Bank Ct.
Orchard Lake, Michigan 48323

ISBN: 0-9660882-0-4

Medical Alternatives Press
4173 Fieldbrook
West Bloomfield, Michigan 48323
(248) 851-3372
(888) 647-5616

Acknowledgements

I gratefully acknowledge the help I have received from my friends and colleagues in putting this book together. This book could not have been published without help from the editors—my wife Allison, Kristin Babcock, Ruth Brownstein, Robert Levine, Jeffrey Nusbaum, Robert Radtke, Jennifer Schafer, Howard Schubiner, Lawrence Schwartz, Adrienne Selko, Shirley Selko and Susana Stoica.

I would also like to thank the following people for assistance in working with the computer graphics in this book: Sonny Benson, Ken Elman, Don Hartlieb, Robert Levine, Scott Lubliner, Marina Mitchell and Susana Stoica.

I would also like to thank my patients. It is your search for natural treatments that are safe and effective that is the driving force behind holistic medicine.

In addition, I cannot thank enough two doctors who helped me realize the benefit of using natural items to promote health: Dr. Stacey Francis and Dr. Robert Radtke.

Update to the 3rd Edition

A special thanks to my editor, Jan Darnell for tirelessly correcting my punctuation. Thanks Jan.

A Word of Caution To The Reader

The information presented in this book is based on the training and professional experience of the author. The treatments recommended in this book should not be undertaken without first consulting a physician. Proper laboratory and clinical monitoring is essential to achieving the goals of finding safe and natural treatments. This book was written for informational and educational purposes only. It is not intended to be used as medical advice.

ABOUT THE AUTHOR

David Brownstein, M.D. is a Board-Certified family physician who utilizes the best of conventional and alternative therapies. He is the Medical Director for the Center for Holistic Medicine in West Bloomfield, MI. He is a graduate of the University of Michigan and Wayne State University School of Medicine. Dr. Brownstein is a member of the American Academy of Family Physicians and the American College for the Advancement in Medicine. He is the father of two beautiful girls, Hailey and Jessica, and is a retired soccer coach. Dr. Brownstein has lectured internationally about his success using natural items. Dr. Brownstein has authored 11 books: _**Iodine: Why You Need It, Why You Can't Live Without It**_, _**Drugs That Don't Work and Natural Therapies That Do, The Miracle of Natural Hormones 3**_rd _**Edition, Overcoming Thyroid Disorders, Overcoming Arthritis, Salt Your Way to Health, The Guide To Healthy Eating, The Guide to a Dairy-Free Diet, The Soy Deception, The Guide to a Gluten-Free Diet**_ and _**Vitamin B12 for Health.**_

Dr. Brownstein's office is located at:

Center for Holistic Medicine
5821 W. Maple Rd.
Ste. 192
West Bloomfield, MI 48323
248.851.1600
www.drbrownstein.com
www.centerforholisticmedicine.com

PREFACE

David Brownstein's *The Miracle of Natural Hormones* is an important and timely book. It addresses an area of medicine that is of central importance in preventive medicine and which is almost universally ignored or grossly mismanaged in conventional medicine. Regrettably, even the practitioners of integrative medicine rarely do justice to this subject. Dr. Brownstein has devoted extraordinary energy to the matter of clinical uses of natural hormone therapies in preserving health and reversing chronic disease, and the result is most commendable. I thank him for writing this book and encourage all integrative physicians to learn well the core messages of this book.

In synthetic hormones we have unleashed a monster. In many synthetic chemicals and pesticides that mimic synthetic hormones in their actions, we have let loose other menacing threats to human biology in general and hormone systems in particular. The monster of synthetic hormones not only interfere with normal hormonal receptors, they also cause serious deficiencies of the body's own natural hormones, which the body needs for maintaining health. This is where Dr. Brownstein's contributions to therapies with natural thyroid hormone, DHEA, natural estrogens, natural testosterone, human growth hormone and melatonin are so valuable.

As we enter the millennium, we should not only take pride in the achievements of modern science and technology, we should also recognize some fundamental and enduring principles of good medicine. Most physicians practicing conventional medicine do not understand the basic concept that injured tissues heal with nutrients and not with drugs. Synthetic hormones are prescribed freely in drug medicine without regard to the basic facts of human biology, the natural cell membrane receptors for hormones evolved with natural hormones and cannot adapt to synthetic molecules. Herein lies the principal danger of synthetic hormones. Forty years ago, as a medical student I learned that one in fifty Pakistani women would probably develop breast cancer. Some years later, as a young surgeon in England, I learned that one in twenty British women might develop breast cancer. A few years later, as a pathologist in the United States, I learned that one in fifteen American women may develop breast cancer. During three decades of my pathology work, the estimated incidence of breast cancer changed from one in fifteen to one in twelve, to one in eleven, to one in ten, to one in nine and to one in eight. In some parts of Long Island, New York, the figure now is one in seven. It is my sad prediction that the number may change to one in five within 30-50 years. I believe the epidemic of breast cancer, as well as that of prostate cancer is due to a synthetic hormonal avalanche that we all face. This avalanche stems from environmental agents as well as prescribing practices of conventional physicians.

One of the mysteries of conventional medicine is how it can claim a synthetic hormone will out-perform a natural hormone. The human body has receptors for natural hormones. No such receptors exist for synthetic hormones. Why does any physician limit himself to prescribing synthetic hormones when natural ones are readily available? The answer, of course, is that mainstream doctors prescribe hormones as drug companies tell them to (through their hired professors). For those doctors as well as practitioners of the new evolving integrative medicine, Dr. Brownstein has done a great service. Using his own case studies, he amply illustrates again and again how natural hormones can effectively be used to preserve health and reverse chronic disease.

David Brownstein is a kind and humanistic practicing physician and that shows well in *The Miracle of Natural Hormones*. He describes his many patients for whom synthetic drugs failed and yet they improved dramatically when they began taking natural hormones. This book includes some rare insights. I whole-heartedly recommend this book to all physicians interested in preventive and integrative medicines.

Majid Ali, M.D.
President and Professor of Medicine
Capital University of Integrative Medicine, Washington, D.C..
Editor, The Journal of Integrative Medicine
Author of the Life Span Library of the Scientific Basis of Health
     The Crab and the Other Side of Cancer
     The Canary and Chronic Fatigue
     RDA: Rats, Drugs and Assumptions
     What Do Lions Know About Stress
     Healing, Miracles and the Bite of the Gray Dog
     The Butterfly and Life Span Nutrition
     The Ghorraa Limbic Exercise
     The Cortical Monkey and Healing

What Others Are Saying About
The Miracle of Natural Hormones

"For the internist, a must read that provides food for thought for the perplexing illnesses that plague our patients. A must read for patients to understand that there are effective natural treatments available to treat many chronic conditions."

Alan Bain, D.O.

"This is for the person who wants to take responsibility for their health. Educate yourself. You must read this book."

Stacey Francis, D.C.

"This book reveals the secrets of optimum health both physically and emotionally. The case studies show how natural hormone replacement can help reverse widespread illness."

Jeffrey Nusbaum, M.D.

"In this book, Dr. Brownstein has truly shown us the future of medicine. Natural hormones have tremendous potential for optimizing health and improving function. This book will surely inspire people and their doctors to include natural hormones in promoting better health."

David Goldstein, M.D.

"Dr. Brownstein's illuminating case histories are presented with state of the art clinical science. The value of this combination derives from his astute empirical observation coupled with a 'health first' paradigm that is modeled after nature herself. By allowing us to recognize our needs, these stories empower us to use natural hormones with gratifying results."

Robert Radtke, D.C.

Dedication

To the women of my life:
Allison, Hailey and Jessica, with all my love.

Contents

Chapter 1

Introduction

Introduction

It has been five years since I wrote the first edition of *The Miracle of Natural Hormones* and I am more convinced than ever of the benefits of using natural hormones. Since that time, none of the statements presented in the first edition (or the second edition) have proven to be false. In fact, recent studies (e.g., The Women's Health Initiative) have pointed out the failure of relying on synthetic hormones to treat illness and promote health. Conversely, other studies have shown the effectiveness of using natural hormones to treat illness and promote optimal health. This book will update those studies and provide new information on the benefits of using natural hormones.

Since the first edition of *The Miracle of Natural Hormones* was published in 1998, I have heard from readers, patients, and physicians of the success they have found with using natural hormones. Although conventional medicine is slow to change, there has been a growing interest in using natural hormones, primarily due to the failure of conventional hormone replacement therapy as reported in the Women's Health Initiative (see Chapter 2). This book will describe the conditions where natural hormones have shown effectiveness and show why natural hormones are so much safer and have a greater efficacy than their synthetic counterparts.

The 21st century presents a challenging time for physicians and patients alike. One day, headlines in the newspapers proclaim the effectiveness of conventional hormones in treating Alzheimer's disease, heart disease, osteoporosis, etc. The next day, different headlines claim that conventional hormones may not help the above conditions and may actually worsen them.

What is the doctor and what is the patient to do?

For the doctor, it is essential to search for an underlying cause(s) of illness and to prescribe treatments that help promote healing and that strengthen the immune system.

For the patient, it is necessary to become knowledgeable about different treatment options available. Patients need to educate themselves about the prescription drugs they use and about the natural items they use. The more involved the patient is in their health care decisions, the better outcome they will receive.

In the 21st century, the scope and complexity of chronic medical conditions plaguing our society is breathtaking-- fibromyalgia, lupus, multiple sclerosis, Crohn's disease, ulcerative colitis, migraine headaches, chronic fatigue syndrome, cancer, osteoporosis, etc. All too often, the treatments proposed by conventional medicine are so toxic that the "cure" is worse than the illness—just ask anyone who has been on long-term steroids to treat some of the above conditions. In order to treat any illness, it is necessary to understand the underlying cause of the illness. If you don't understand the underlying cause of the illness, then how can you develop an effective treatment plan?

As a society, we have settled for sub-par health. People who suffer from chronic fatigue syndrome are often told by their physicians, "There is no treatment, you just have to live with it." Those who suffer from headaches, including migraine headaches, are often given medicines that have side effects worse than the headache itself. If one medication doesn't work, there is always another one to take its place. Many times, these medications only treat the symptoms of disease, they do not address the underlying cause of the illness.

This book will show you that often times the underlying cause of many chronic illnesses may be a hormonal imbalance. It is impossible to achieve your optimal health without first achieving balance within the hormonal system. All of the systems of the body, including the nervous system, the cardiovascular system, the immune system and the circulatory system depend upon a balanced hormonal system.

I have found that the clinical use of natural hormones restores hormonal imbalance. Natural hormones can be an effective treatment option not only for promoting optimal health but also for treating many chronic illnesses including; chronic fatigue syndrome, fibromyalgia, PMS, heart disease, menopausal symptoms, autoimmune disorders and many other conditions.

A hormone is a chemical substance produced in the body by a gland. Hormones have a specific regulatory effect on the activity of the body. For example, the thyroid gland produces thyroid hormone and thyroid hormone helps regulate the metabolism of the body.

Natural hormones are substances generally produced from plant products that closely mimic the body's own hormone production, both structurally and chemically. Examples of natural hormones covered in this book include desiccated thyroid, DHEA, natural progesterone, natural estrogens, natural testosterone, melatonin, hydrocortisone, human growth hormone and pregnenolone. Hormones that have been chemically altered are termed synthetic hormones.

Synthetic hormones are not naturally occurring substances in the body. In fact, synthetic hormones are not found in any living forms. Synthetic hormones can be thought of as foreign substances to the body. Because they are foreign substances to the body, is there any wonder that there are so many serious side effects with the use of synthetic hormones? Examples of synthetic hormones include Provera, birth control pills, etc.

Hormones work in our bodies via a "lock and key"' model. When a hormone is released from its gland the hormone (the "key") binds to its receptor (the "lock"). This binding is analogous to a key being put in the ignition of the car. When the binding occurs a chemical reaction takes place. Natural hormones have a perfect fit in these receptors. The "key" fits perfectly in its complimentary "lock". This is contrasted with a synthetic hormone in which the un-natural hormone (i.e., the "key") does not fit well in the body's receptor (i.e., the "lock"). This un-natural fit results in the high rate of adverse effects seen with the use of synthetic hormones. A comparison of the chemical structure of a natural hormone (natural progesterone) and a synthetic hormone (Provera) is shown in Figure 7 (page 97). I believe that if we are going to use a hormone to treat any condition, we should use a natural hormone over a synthetic hormone every time.

Natural hormones, when used appropriately, will enhance one's health and will treat or even cure diseases, all without any appreciable side effects. Many physicians erroneously believe there is no difference between a synthetic hormone and a natural hormone. That is usually because these physicians have little or no experience in the use of natural hormones and other natural products. My clinical experience shows that there is no better substitute for the body's own production of hormones than using a natural form of that hormone. This experience has been repeatedly confirmed by my patients' positive responses to natural hormones.

Natural hormones can improve well-being, slow aging and reverse many chronic conditions. After taking natural hormones, my older patients constantly proclaim that they feel like they did when they were in their 20's. I have found natural hormones to be a great benefit and often a cure for many conditions including;

chronic fatigue syndrome, PMS, endometriosis, infertility, headaches and migraine headaches, recurrent infections, fibromyalgia, ulcerative colitis, Crohn's, and other autoimmune disorders. It is rare for a patient with any of the above conditions not to show significant improvement in their conditions after taking natural hormones. I am continually amazed at how many chronic diseases can be halted and, many times, cured through the use of natural hormones.

My patients are familiar with the following question: "If it is found that you are low in a hormone, and you are given a choice of a natural hormone—one that closely mimics your own hormone chemically and structurally, versus a synthetic hormone—a man-made derivative of a hormone that has been structurally altered to become a patentable product, which one would you pick?" A vast scientific knowledge base is not needed to realize a natural hormone will perform better than a synthetic hormone every time.

Man has searched for a fountain of youth for thousands of years. Although there is no "cure" for aging, my clinical experience has shown that natural hormones, when used appropriately, can slow down many of the signs of aging including deteriorating mental function, loss of muscle tone, and wrinkled skin. Hormone production peaks when we are young, usually in the age range from 20 to 30. In older people, supplementation with natural hormones can reverse many of the signs of aging. Synthetic hormones do not provide the same anti-aging benefit as natural hormones.

This statement holds true when comparing all natural products to synthetic products, including vitamins, minerals and herbs. It is a common-sense argument to use a natural product to treat disease and promote health, and there are many studies that back up this idea.

Many patients are on synthetic hormones when they first come to my office. Often, just changing them over to natural hormones dramatically improves their condition. Dennis, a 52-year-old CEO of a manufacturing company, had been on Synthroid, a synthetic thyroid hormone, for 10 years. He complained that he always felt lethargic and had aching muscles, cold limbs, and dry skin. He was also being treated for hypertension with Procardia, a common antihypertensive medication. His lab work indicated normal thyroid levels. After taking Armour thyroid hormone for one month, Dennis reported feeling 80% better overall. This story repeats itself over and over in my practice. Dr. Alan Gaby, a pioneering physician in natural therapies, wrote in the Journal of the American Medical Association of his similar experience with symptom improvements in patients after switching them from synthetic thyroid preparations to a natural version.

Natural hormones work better when used in combinations. When I see books about individual natural hormones such as DHEA, I find the fault of these theories is they only address one hormone at a time. My experience shows that this is not the correct approach. A chronic condition is often a sign of a serious imbalance in the immune system of the body. This imbalance usually cannot be successfully treated with a single agent. In order to bring the immune system into a more balanced state, combinations of therapies are often necessary. I have found using combinations of natural hormones, when indicated, can often reverse this imbalance and even cure many chronic diseases. I have not had nearly as much success in my practice using natural hormones individually to treat disease or to slow down the signs of aging.

I have chosen to talk about the natural hormones separately. However, I cannot emphasize enough that the greatest benefit of these hormones is achieved when they are used in combination with each other. These hormones have a synergistic effect with one another.

The natural hormones described in this book are used only in "physiologic doses." A physiologic dose of a natural hormone refers to a small enough dose so as not to cause the body to cease production of the hormone. When hormones are given in "pharmacologic doses," (i.e., doses larger than the normal production in the body), the body senses an overload of that particular hormone and will cease all production of it. Many problems attributed to hormones- for example, body builders getting cancer and other side effects from using too much testosterone- can be attributed to using excess or large pharmacologic doses. I have observed no serious side effects from any of the natural hormones covered in this book when physiologic doses are used.

All of the natural treatments described in this book should be managed with a health care provider—someone knowledgeable in the use of natural hormones. The hormones covered in this book can significantly help chronic conditions, improve health, and slow down the signs of aging. However, they can also harm you if not used appropriately and under the guidance of a knowledgeable health care provider. Improved results are achieved when other natural agents, such as vitamins, minerals, and herbs, are used to support these hormones.

Chapter 2

The Failure of Conventional HRT: The Women's Health Study Initiative

Introduction

The Women's Health Initiative (WHI) was designed to provide information about the risks and benefits of conventional hormone replacement therapy. The WHI was a study involving 40 large medical centers around the United States, with 16,608 women. The WHI began in 1996 and was reported in July, 2002.

The WHI was a randomized, placebo controlled study. This means that half of the women received conventional hormone replacement in the form of Prempro (Premarin and Provera) and half received a placebo (no active drug).

The outcomes the researchers were looking for included increases or decreases in breast cancer, heart disease, stroke, pulmonary embolism, colorectal cancer, endometrial cancer, hip fracture and death due to any cause.

The study was supposed to last 8.5 years. The researchers halted the study at 5.2 years because the overall risks of conventional hormone replacement therapy outweighed the overall benefits. This Chapter will review the risks and benefits reported in WHI, and correlate these findings to previous studies on hormone replacement therapy.

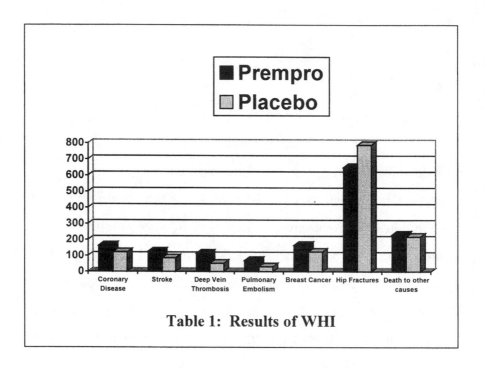

Table 1: Results of WHI

Results of WHI: The Good

Table 1 shows the results of the WHI. There were positive outcomes reported from WHI. There was a 21% decrease in osteoporotic fractures in the Prempro group as compared to the placebo group. In addition, there was a 37% decrease in colorectal cancer in the Prempro group.

Results of WHI: The Bad

There was a 29% increase in coronary heart disease in the Prempro group.

Results of WHI: The Ugly

A 41% increase in stroke and a remarkable 2,100% increase in pulmonary embolism (i.e., lung blood clots) was found in the treated (i.e., Prempro) group. In addition the Prempro group had a 26% increase risk of breast cancer.

The Implications of WHI

The WHI was supposed to be an 8.5-year study. However, the research was stopped early, at 5.2 years, when the authors of the study realized that the risks of conventional hormone replacement therapy outweighed the benefits.

The results of the WHI made national headlines. It was the final blow to the widespread use of conventional hormone replacement therapy. Women were flocking to their doctors asking them what to do with their hormone replacement therapy. The headlines in the newspapers across the country suggested that important, new information had come to light on the use of conventional hormones.

Since the WHI made such an impact nationwide, the question to ask is: What were the new findings in the WHI that made so many women (and their physicians) question the benefits of taking conventional hormone replacement therapy?

The answer to the above question can be summed up in one word: **nothing**. There was no new information in the WHI that wasn't already available in the past. In fact many other studies had already shown the negative influences conventional hormone replacement therapy had on cardiovascular disease, strokes and other blood clots as well as cancer.

Coronary Artery Disease

In a landmark article in 1998, researchers reported increased cardiovascular events in the conventional hormone treated group as compared to a controlled group that took a placebo.[1] The American Heart Association came out against using conventional hormone replacement therapy for the sole reason of preventing future heart attacks.[2] An article in the New England Journal of Medicine cited similar results showing conventional hormone replacement therapy ineffective for preventing heart disease.[3]

The Women's Health Initiative research study showed a 29% increase in cardiovascular disease in the group that took Prempro. This study confirmed the earlier studies on the ineffectiveness of conventional hormone replacement therapy in preventing cardiovascular disease.

In addition, WHI showed that there was no benefit for stroke prevention. Instead, women who took conventional hormones had a 41% increased risk of stroke compared to women who did not take the hormones. It is even more alarming that a 2,100% increased risk for pulmonary embolism was observed. The increased risk for cardiac events has been reported in many different studies in women who use conventional hormone replacement therapy.

Breast Cancer

Perhaps the greatest downfall of the WHI occurred with the negative findings of breast cancer. The concern with increasing the risk for breast cancer by using conventional hormones has been around for almost 20 years. Many previous studies have shown an increased risk of breast cancer with the use of conventional hormones.[4][5][6][7].

Breast cancer is every woman's fear. It is approaching (if it hasn't already exceeded) epidemic rates in this country. Today, approximately 1 in 7 women in the United States are affected by breast cancer.

With such high rates of breast cancer prevalent today, no therapy should be given that will further increase the rate of breast cancer. The WHI clearly showed that the use of conventional hormones was responsible for a 26% increased risk of breast cancer in women who took conventional hormones. As mentioned above, the WHI was not the first study to point out this increased risk. The studies showing an increased risk of breast cancer date back to the 1980's.

As a physician, I took an oath at my medical school graduation that said in part, "Above all, do no harm". The WHI study, as well as many previous studies, showed that the use of conventional hormones is often harmful. I believe safer methods need to be examined, and this will only occur with the use of bio-identical (i.e., natural) hormones.

Final Thoughts: Natural Hormone Prescribing Doctors Have Been Vindicated

Many physicians who have taken the viewpoint that natural hormones are safer than their synthetic counterparts have been making the claim for years that synthetic hormones are not safe. Those of us that have taken the path less traveled have often been derided by our conventional colleagues for using natural hormones. The arguments conventional physicians often use against using natural hormones include:

1. There are no studies showing the benefits of natural hormones.

2. Natural hormones are not absorbed well.

The argument that there are no studies showing the benefits of natural hormones is false. Although they are not as plentiful, there are many studies showing the benefits of natural hormones (see references in back of this book). This argument (not enough studies) should actually be used for the conventional hormones. I believe that there has never been adequate documentation that synthetic hormones have any appreciable health benefits. How could they, when they act as a foreign substance to the body?

The reason that there is not an abundance of studies on natural hormones is because natural hormones are not patentable items. If a drug company holds a patent on a particular drug, it is interested in publishing research on that drug in order to sell more of it. It is against the law to patent a natural product, like a natural hormone. Therefore, the money to do a proper research study on natural hormones (or any natural product) will not come from a drug company (as they will not hold the patent to the natural product).

Another argument against the use of natural hormones that is often used by conventional physicians is that natural hormones are not well absorbed. This is simply not true. For over 10 years, I have been checking pre and post serum levels of hormones on my patients. The serum levels clearly indicate that there is adequate absorption of natural hormones through a transdermal or oral preparation. On the contrary, there are no reliable tests available to measure the levels of synthetic hormones like Provera and Premarin. Women are generally treated with these synthetic agents without any blood tests. How can you determine the proper dose of a medication if you have no way of monitoring the medication? You can't.

The Women's Health Study Initiative was a vindication for all the physicians who promote the use of natural hormones. It makes perfect sense to use a natural product in the place of a synthetic product, when it is available. Natural hormones are safer and more effective than their synthetic counterparts and they should be employed for all cases that require the use of hormones.

[1] Hulley, Stephen, et al. Randomized trial of estrogen plus progestin for secondary prevention of coronary heart disease in postmenopausal women. JAMA. Vol. 280 No. 7, 8/19/98

[2] Circulation. July 24, 2001;104;459-503

[3] New England Journal of Medicine. 8/24/00;343:522-529

[4] J. Natl. Cancer Inst. 92(4) 328-332, 2000

[5] Menopausal Estrogen and Estrogen-Progestin Replacement Therapy and Breast Cancer Risk. JAMA. 1/26/2000. Vol. 283, No.4

[6] The risk of breast cancer after estrogen and estrogen-progestin replacement. N. Engl. J. Med. 1989;321:293-297

[7] The use of estrogens and progestins and the risk of breast cancer in postmenopausal women. N. Engl. J. Med. 1995;332:1589-1593

Chapter 3

Hypothyroidism

BENEFITS OF THYROID HORMONE

Low thyroid function, known as hypothyroidism, can be treated with thyroid hormone. The symptoms of hypothyroidism include: fatigue, difficulty getting up in the morning, cold extremities and intolerance to cold, dry skin, psoriasis, eczema, acne, recurrent infections, constipation, menstrual disorders, premenstrual syndrome (PMS), infertility, hypercholesterol, atherosclerosis, obesity and difficulty losing weight, hypoglycemia, diminished sweating, brittle nails, poor memory, depression, headaches and migraine headaches, fibrocystic breast disease, ovarian cysts and generalized weakness.

Introduction

The thyroid gland is a butterfly shaped gland located in the lower part of the neck. Though it weighs less than an ounce, the thyroid is responsible for many critical functions in the body. Every single muscle, organ and cell in the body depends on adequate thyroid hormone levels for proper functioning. I have found that even a slight deficiency of thyroid hormone, known as hypothyroidism, can tremendously impact one's health.

The thyroid is the main hormone-producing gland regulating body metabolism and is directly responsible for energy production. Inadequate production of thyroid hormone will lead to other glandular imbalances (i.e., adrenal, ovarian, pituitary, etc.).

Natural thyroid hormone known as desiccated thyroid or Armour thyroid is much more effective for treating hypothyroidism than synthetic versions such as Synthroid or Levothroid. Although Armour thyroid does not exactly mimic the human body's production of thyroid hormone, it is the closest derivative of human thyroid hormone available.

A diagnosis of hypothyroidism should not be made solely on blood tests. An accurate diagnosis should encompass correlating the blood tests along with basal temperatures and physical exam signs and symptoms (explained in the discussion section). All cases studies mentioned in this book had thyroid blood tests performed before treatment. Occasionally, thyroid blood tests do not correlate with other signs of hypothyroidism. This will be more fully clarified in the discussion section. More information on hypothyroidism can be found in my book, *Overcoming Thyroid Disorders*.

Case Studies

Fatigue and Chronic Fatigue Immune Dysfunction Syndrome (CFIDS)

Fatigue is one of the most common complaints that people report to their physician. Fatigue can be a complaint of numerous medical conditions, including anemia, cancer, infections, etc. Fatigue can also be a presenting symptom of hypothyroidism, as long-standing hypothyroidism can lead to long-standing fatigue.

It has been known for over 100 years that thyroid abnormalities can present as a fatigue state. Chronic fatigue immune dysfunction syndrome (CFIDS) strikes over one million Americans.[1] CFIDS is characterized by long-standing (greater than 6 months) fatigue, sore throat, muscle aches, etc. It can affect people of any age, race or socioeconomic status. CFIDS affects women at a rate of 3:1 over men. In the case of CFIDS, my clinical experience has shown that a large percentage of CFIDS patients have hypothyroidism. Researchers have reported relief of CFIDS symptoms when patients were treated with thyroid hormone.[2]

CFIDS is a very difficult condition both to diagnose and treat and many physicians still doubt it truly exists. I see many patients suffering from this illness, only to be told by their physician that there is no treatment available. I have found nearly 100% of my patients with chronic fatigue suffer from hormonal imbalances and many of them are hypothyroid.

Phil, a 32-year-old engineer was diagnosed with chronic fatigue syndrome five years ago. After seeking care from four doctors, he was told nothing could be done to help him. Though Phil was able to work, he had no life outside of work. "I used to enjoy sports, now I barely have the energy to watch sports on television. Furthermore, I am cold all of the time, even when everyone else is complaining how warm it is," Phil declared. Phil's basal body temperature averaged 96.6 degrees Fahrenheit—more than one degree below normal. He drank inordinately large amounts of caffeinated beverages in order to keep him going, but to no avail. When Phil was started on Armour thyroid hormone, he immediately noticed an improvement in his condition. Each time the dose was increased, he noticed a stepwise improvement. It took three months to finally achieve an adequate thyroid level, with two grains of Armour thyroid, whereupon Phil felt as if he had "been reborn." Furthermore, his basal temperature improved to a healthy 98.0 degrees Fahrenheit. Today, two years after starting thyroid hormone, Phil remains symptom free. Good health and a resolution of many conditions like CFIDS is possible with the proper use of natural hormones.

Hetty, 65 years old, had not felt well in over 10 years. "It came on gradually over the years, then I became so fatigued that I could not think straight," she said. Hetty had to go on a medical leave from work because she was so fatigued that she could not think clearly. She said, "My brain felt like it was in a fog." Hetty had seen many doctors and they all told her the same thing: "Nothing is wrong, perhaps you are depressed." Hetty kept insisting that something was wrong with her thyroid gland. When I examined Hetty, she had many of the clinical signs of hypothyroidism including poor eyebrow growth, hair falling out, puffiness of her face, weight gain and low basal body temperatures. However, Hetty's blood tests fell within the *normal range. I felt that Hetty's clinical picture warranted a therapeutic trial of Armour thyroid hormone. "Within one week of starting the thyroid hormone, I started to come out of the fog. I could get out of bed and actually move around without feeling wiped out. I didn't realize how bad I was until I started to feel better," she said. Now, five years later, Hetty is still taking Armour thyroid hormone. She has improved so much that she presently works in my office.*

Hetty's case illustrates how the blood tests may not tell the whole story. I believe it is necessary to correlate the blood tests with the basal body temperatures (see Figure 1, page 41) and the clinical signs and symptoms. This is a holistic way to diagnose a systemic illness like hypothyroidism.

Headaches and Migraine Headaches

I have found that many individuals who suffer from headaches, including migraine headaches, often have a thyroid problem. Conventional medicine has little to offer headache sufferers. The medications used to treat headaches primarily treat the symptoms of the headache; they do not treat the underlying cause(s). I used to find headache and migraine headache patients frustrating to treat because I could rarely provide long-term relief; often I could only help with symptom relief. I have found that the correction of a hormonal imbalance, particularly a thyroid imbalance, is very effective at significantly improving and sometimes curing headaches.

Mary, a 46-year-old teacher, complained, "I have a headache every day of my life." Coupled with her daily headaches, she would sometimes suffer with up to two migraine headaches per week. The only thing Mary could do to control them was to take Imitrex, a prescription medication commonly used to treat migraines. "The Imitrex was almost worse than the headache," Mary complained. Mary was missing work two to three days per month due to her headaches. Mary was prescribed numerous headache medicines and almost all of them made her feel worse. In addition to the constant headaches, Mary had other symptoms typical of people suffering from hypothyroidism including always having cold hands and feet. "I'm always cold, and my husband won't let me touch him because my hands and feet feel like they came out of the refrigerator," Mary said. She also suffered from constipation and had daily achiness in her joints and muscles. She commented, "Because I'm always stiff, I feel like I'm 80 years old." One measure of how the thyroid is functioning is to measure the body's temperature at rest, also known as the basal body temperature. A normal basal body temperature averages 97.8-98.2 degrees Fahrenheit and is explained in the Discussion section on page 41. Mary's basal temperature averaged 97.2 degrees Fahrenheit and her blood tests indicated a hypothyroid state. Mary was placed on 60mg of Armour thyroid hormone and returned one month later. Mary was pleased at her progress and said, "I did not realize how depressed I was until now. For the last three or four years, it was an effort to do anything. After the first week of taking the thyroid medication, my headaches just stopped. I couldn't believe it. Also, my bowels started working better and my achiness is almost totally gone. In addition, I have become a much better teacher because my energy level is so much better." After five months on Armour thyroid, all of Mary's symptoms resolved. She was happy to report, "I feel like I have lost 20 years of aging since beginning the thyroid therapy. I feel as good as I did when I was in my 20's."

Jordan, a 37-year-old family physician was frustrated with his migraine headaches. "I have tried all the known prescription medications and none of them helped. My headaches are getting worse, occurring sometimes two times per week. I'm afraid I am going to have to cut back on seeing patients if I cannot control these headaches," he lamented. Jordan had also been taking antihypertensive medications since he was 16 years old. He complained of being constantly cold, especially having cold hands and feet. Jordan stated, "My patients cringe when I touch them because my hands feel like ice." In addition, he reported feeling fatigued and having a difficult time concentrating. "I used to love reading novels. Now, I find it extremely difficult to read any long books because I cannot concentrate for extended periods of time," he stated. Hypothyroid individuals will often find their mental capacities diminished. Proper levels of thyroid hormone are extremely important for maintaining proper cognitive abilities.

Jordan's basal temperature averaged 96.8 degrees Fahrenheit. Upon taking Armour thyroid hormone, Jordan noticed an immediate improvement. One month later he reported his headaches were 50% better. Six months later his headaches were almost completely gone. "I can't believe it. My headaches just melted away with the thyroid hormone. I also have more energy and I am much more focused during the day. My ability to concentrate has returned to normal and I have started to enjoy reading again," he said. Jordan's blood pressure also improved on the thyroid therapy, and he was able to cut the dosage of his anti-hypertensive medication in half. "I have started to look more closely at evaluating my patients for thyroid problems and I now have all my patients check their basal temperatures," Jordan reported.

Sally, a 48-year-old physical therapist, also suffered from headaches. Her headaches began at age 25 when she had a hysterectomy with removal of her ovaries for severe endometriosis—a painful condition where uterine tissue grows outside of the uterus in the pelvic cavity. She was placed on Premarin, a synthetic estrogen hormone, and reported, "I never felt good after the surgery. I traded one set of problems—terribly painful periods and heavy bleeding—for constant headaches and migraine headaches." She also complained of always feeling fatigued, being cold all the time, and having high cholesterol levels (250mg/dl). In addition, she had developed numerous food and environmental allergies, especially to dogs and cats, over the past three years. "I feel like I am falling apart," she said. Her physical exam revealed poor eyebrow growth and a very thickened tongue, which are both consistent with a hypothyroid condition. Her thyroid blood tests were in the low range of normal and her basal temperature averaged 97.0 degrees Fahrenheit. After taking Armour thyroid, she noticed an immediate improvement. At her one-month checkup, Sally reported a 75% overall improvement, with her headaches reduced to a "minor annoyance." At a two-month check-up, she was no longer experiencing any migraine headaches. Furthermore, her energy level had significantly improved. "I feel like I am alive again," she commented at that visit. Eventually, DHEA (covered in Chapter 5) and natural progesterone (covered in Chapter 6) were added due to low serum levels. Shortly after beginning treatment, Sally reported feeling 100% improved. At a four-month visit, Sally exclaimed, "It truly is a miracle. I didn't know I could ever feel this good." All signs of Sally's fatigue and headaches resolved. Sally returned for her six-month checkup, and reported her allergy symptoms were almost totally gone. "My kids cannot believe I can now be around dogs and cats. I tried allergy shots for 10 years and have taken allergy pills twice a day for 15 years. I don't take anything now and my allergy symptoms are gone." I have observed many patients' allergy symptoms improve when their hypothyroid condition is addressed with the use of Armour thyroid hormone.

Poor Recovery From Infection

When hypothyroid people become ill, they often find it difficult, if not impossible, to fully recover from their illness. The body's primary defense against infections is the immune system. Many factors lower the immune system's level of functioning, such as lack of sleep, stress, and poor nutrition. Likewise, it is impossible to have an adequately functioning immune system without proper thyroid functioning. Hypothyroid people will often report getting every viral illness that comes around, as well as being unable to fully recover from infection.

Molly, age 32, was well until two years ago, when she contacted malaria while working as a safari tour guide in Africa. "I had malaria for three weeks and I have never fully recovered. I used to have all the energy in the world, now I can't do anything. I can't even hold down a job. It is a great effort for me just to get through the day. My energy level feels like it is totally depleted," she lamented. She also reported being constipated and cold all the time, and having extremely cold hands and feet. "I have to sleep with socks even during most of the summer," she said. Molly went from doctor to doctor only to be told that her blood tests were normal, indicating nothing was wrong. She was given a trial of antidepressant drugs to no avail. When she questioned an internist on how she could feel so bad and have nothing wrong, she was told to have her husband buy her a fur coat to make her feel better. Molly's basal temperature averaged 96.4 degrees Fahrenheit. Upon taking Armour thyroid hormone, Molly's temperature rose to a normal level of 98.0 degrees Fahrenheit. Most importantly, all her symptoms began improving. At a six-week check-up, she reported, "I can't believe how good I feel. I am starting to feel like my old self again. I used to have to take a nap every day, now I can get through the whole day without a nap and feel good. Since taking the Armour thyroid hormone, my friends tell me I look younger and they want to know what I am doing." I see many people in my practice who report they were well until they had a minor illness from which they have not been able to recover. This failure to fully recover from an infection can be a sign of a thyroid problem. Hypothyroidism should be investigated in anyone who has difficulty completely recovering from an illness, as well as someone who constantly suffers from recurrent infections.

Infertility

Hypothyroidism is often an overlooked diagnosis for infertility problems. I have found that many infertility patients, both women and men, respond favorably to natural thyroid hormone replacement therapy. Adequate thyroid hormone secretion is necessary for the development of the egg, proper ovarian function and having regular menstrual cycles with ovulation. I believe many infertile couples could be spared the expense and agony of the inability to conceive by having their thyroid gland properly evaluated.

Heather, a 32-year-old accounting executive had spent $30,000 trying to get pregnant with high-tech infertility treatments *such as in vitro fertilization, all without success. In addition, she underwent severe emotional mood swings from using powerful drugs to try and stimulate her ovaries to ovulate. "Emotionally I can't go through those procedures anymore. I had tremendous mood swings on those drugs and I couldn't stand the way the drugs made me act. I can't take those drugs again,' she stated. In addition to infertility, Heather was always fatigued, constipated, had irregular and painful menstrual periods and felt cold all of the time. "Even when everyone else at work is hot, I complain about how cold it is. I have to wear long underwear to work for most of the year just to stay warm," she lamented. Heather's blood tests revealed a borderline hypothyroid state, but her basal temperatures averaged 96.5 degrees Fahrenheit—more than one degree below normal. Upon placing her on Armour thyroid hormone, all of her symptoms rapidly improved. Heather became pregnant four months later and delivered a healthy eight-pound baby boy.*

I have seen many cases of infertility "spontaneously" cured when hypothyroidism is properly diagnosed and treated. It is well known in the medical literature that hypothyroidism predisposes one to an infertile state. I believe that before resorting to toxic hormonal therapies to treat infertility, a complete workup of the thyroid gland should be undertaken. Dr. Broda O. Barnes, a pioneer in the diagnosis and treatment of hypothyroidism wrote of his success in using thyroid hormone to treat infertility problems over 25 years ago.[3]

Sherri, a 34-year-old teacher, had been unable to conceive for two years. She had been seeing an infertility doctor and was treated with drugs, including Clomid, to help her ovulate. Sherri claimed, "Each month, the stress on me gets greater and greater. My infertility doctor cannot explain why I cannot get pregnant. My marriage has suffered throughout all this and my husband and I constantly fight now." In addition to not being able to get pregnant, Sherri complained of always being fatigued, having cold hands and feet, having very dry skin and intermittent hair loss. In addition, she suffered from severe premenstrual mood swings. "No one can stand to be around me for the week before my period. I seem angry at the world during this time," she stated. All of her symptoms were consistent with a hypothyroid state. When I reviewed Sherri's basal temperatures, which she had been tracking to monitor her infertility workup, I was not surprised to see a low basal temperature. Her basal temperature averaged 96.6 degrees Fahrenheit—more than one degree below normal. When Sherri started taking Armour thyroid hormone, all of her symptoms began to improve rapidly. After three months on Armour thyroid hormone, Sherri reported, "I've never felt better in my whole life. My husband and I are getting along much better. We don't seem to fight anymore." At this point, she stopped the infertility drugs because she did not like the mood swings they caused. Shortly thereafter, Sherri became pregnant and delivered a healthy nine-pound baby boy. Two years later, Sherri had no problem becoming pregnant again and she now has two healthy baby boys.

Poor Response To Levothyroxine (Synthroid, Levothroid or Unithroid)

Barbara, a 62-year-old school principal, came to me with complaints of fatigue for 10 years, difficulty concentrating, cold hands and feet, constipation, hair loss, high cholesterol levels (265mg/dl), frequent infections and fibrocystic breasts. Barbara had been taking Synthroid for 10 years and reported, "It never did a thing for me." After doing some research, Barbara recently went to an endocrinologist and told him she thought the Synthroid was not working correctly. As she was listing off the above problems, he sat there and shook his head 'no' to her. Barbara stated, "He frequently interrupted me to tell me my blood tests were normal, indicating this was not a thyroid problem. When I asked what the problem was, he told me I was depressed and needed an antidepressant. I knew I didn't feel well, but something was wrong and it was not from depression." Barbara's basal temperature averaged 96.6 degrees Fahrenheit, over one degree lower than normal, indicating that she was not responding to Synthroid. Upon placing her on Armour thyroid hormone, all her symptoms improved dramatically within six weeks. "It amazes me that I was taking a thyroid hormone that wasn't doing anything for me. Now that I am feeling so much better, I realize how sick I was and I can see how much thyroid hormone has to do with health," she said at her follow-up visit. All of Barbara's symptoms improved on Armour thyroid, and her cholesterol fell to a normal 196ng/dl four months later.

Synthroid and Levothroid are relatively inactive forms of thyroid hormone. Armour thyroid contains a much more active form of thyroid hormone. My clinical experience has consistently shown most patients generally do much better on Armour thyroid rather than Synthroid or Levothroid. This will be explained more in the Discussion section.

Seizure Disorders

Ethan, 9 years old, was born eight weeks premature. He was in the hospital for 10 weeks after he was born because of a seizure disorder. When I saw Ethan three years ago, he was still having three to four seizures per month, even though he was on high doses of anti-seizure medications. When I fist saw Ethan, I was struck by his appearance. Ethan's face was extremely puffy. His tongue was so large it was protruding out of his mouth. He had very poor tone in his muscles and his reflexes were slow. In addition, his hair was very thin and he had minimal eyebrow growth. All of these clinical signs are consistent with a hypothyroid state. Ethan's basal temperature averaged 96.0 degrees Fahrenheit and his blood work indicated a hypothyroid condition. Ethan responded immediately to small amounts of Armour thyroid hormone. All of his clinical signs improved, and he has yet to have a seizure since taking his first thyroid dose. Furthermore, he has been able to significantly decrease the dose of his anti-seizure mediation. Recently, Ethan's mother sent me a note saying that because of the Armour thyroid hormone, it has been over 2 years since Ethan has had a seizure.

I have had many similar experiences with thyroid hormone replacement significantly reducing or eliminating seizure disorders in adults as well as children. A normal functioning thyroid gland is necessary for the proper development and maintenance of the nervous system. Anyone with a neurological disorder should have their thyroid gland properly evaluated to rule out a hypothyroid condition.

Discussion

The thyroid is responsible for the body's metabolism and the production of heat. Hypothyroid individuals will often report being cold or having cold hands and feet. One measure of how the thyroid is performing can be ascertained with a $2.00 instrument. This 'medical' device is a basal thermometer, available at a local pharmacy. I advise my patients to check their basal temperature routinely. Though it should not be the sole measurement in the diagnosis of thyroid abnormalities, it is very useful. The instructions for taking basal body temperatures are illustrated on page 41.

The thyroid gland produces the hormone thyroxine, commonly known as T4. T4 is an inactive form of thyroid hormone in the body. In order for T4 to be activated in the body, it is converted to a more active hormone—Triiodothyronine, known as T3. T3 is the 'activated' form of thyroid hormone that exerts its influences on all the cells of the body (see Figure 2). For treatment of low thyroid function, I recommend using natural desiccated thyroid hormone, most commonly known as Armour thyroid, instead of synthetic thyroid preparations such as Synthroid, Levothyroxine or Unithroid.

Figure 1: How to Measure the Basal Body Temperature

1. Shake down a basal thermometer the night before and place at your bedside. If you don't have a basal thermometer, a digital thermometer is adequate.
2. Upon awakening, place the thermometer snugly in your armpit for a period of 10 minutes and record your temperature for 5 days in a row. You must not get out of bed before checking your temperature or you will have an altered reading.
3. For women who are menstruating, the temperature should be taken starting on the second day of menstruation. This is the best time in a woman's menstrual cycle to get an accurate basal temperature. For men and postmenopausal women, it makes no difference when the temperatures are taken.
4. If your thyroid function is normal, your temperature should be in the range of 97.8-98.2 degrees Fahrenheit. A temperature below this may indicate a hypothyroid state.
5. If you are taking the temperatures orally, your temperature should be in the range of 98.8-99.2 degrees Fahrenheit. A temperature below this may indicate a hypothyroid state.

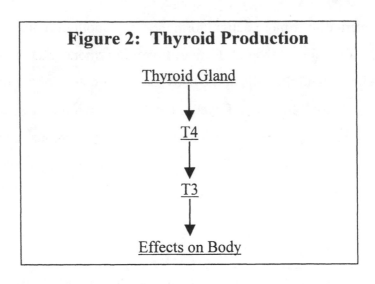

Figure 2: Thyroid Production

Thyroid Gland

T4

T3

Effects on Body

Desiccated thyroid is a porcine thyroid preparation, containing both T4 and T3, in proportions very close to the natural human thyroid output. Also, it has other factors that more readily allow for the conversion of T4 to the active form T3. Synthetic thyroid preparations such as Synthroid or Levothyroxine, contain only T4 thyroid hormone, which has to be converted to T3 in the body to be effective. Although Armour thyroid hormone does not exactly mimic the human thyroid production, it is the closest natural thyroid hormone presently available.

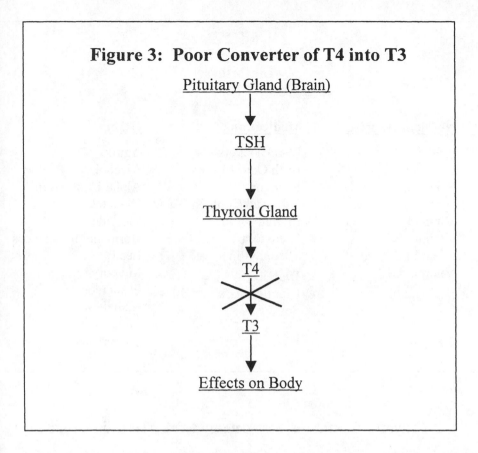

Figure 3: Poor Converter of T4 into T3

Pituitary Gland (Brain)

TSH

Thyroid Gland

T4

T3

Effects on Body

Many people fail to respond to synthetic T4 preparations like Synthroid, because they cannot adequately convert the T4 to the active form—T3 (see Figure 3). As a result, they will get a sub-optimal response to synthetic preparations. I see this problem occurring in those patients that report little or no improvement from taking synthetic preparations. Many of these patients will improve upon taking Amour thyroid. Many factors may be responsible for the inability of the body to convert thyroid hormone to a more active form as shown in Table 1.

Table 1: T4 to T3 Inhibitors

Nutrient Deficiencies	Medications	Other
Iodine	Beta Blockers	Aging
Iron	Birth Control Pills	Alcohol
Selenium	Estrogen	Alpha-Lipoic Acid
Zinc	Iodinated Contrast Agent	Diabetes
Vitamin A	Lithium	Fluoride
Vitamin B2	Phenytoin	Hormonal Imbalances
Vitamin B6	Theophylline	Lead
Vitamin B12	**Diet**	Mercury
	Cruciferous Vegetables	Pesticides
	Soy	Radiation
		Stress
		Surgery

Thyroid function is best determined by correlating one's health history, clinical examination, conventional blood testing and serial monitoring of basal temperatures. Conventional medicine primarily relies on blood testing to make the diagnosis of hypothyroidism, regardless of the patient's condition or clinical symptoms. In fact, many patients' complaints are virtually ignored by conventional doctors if their blood tests for thyroid function indicate normal values. This is where the problem lies. I have evaluated and treated patients for hypothyroidism who have normal blood work. Many times these patients had every clinical sign present to make a diagnosis of hypothyroidism such as fatigue, a sense of coldness including having extremely cold hands and feet, constipation, high cholesterol levels, headaches, hair falling out, dry skin, acne, etc. These clinical signs were correlated with low basal body temperatures, which in hypothyroid individuals will typically run below 97.4 degrees Fahrenheit. Most of these patients will improve and their clinical symptoms will abate almost immediately when they are placed on small amounts of Armour thyroid hormone. In addition, their basal temperature will increase into the normal range of 97.8-98.2 degrees Fahrenheit.

Why would the blood test fail to detect a low thyroid state? Thyroid hormone exerts its influence on the body at the cellular level, which is the deepest level in the body. Thyroid blood tests do not indicate the cellular level function. In fact, there is no test available that indicates the cellular influence of thyroid hormone.

Thyroid Hormone Resistance

Another reason the blood tests may not reveal the actual functioning of thyroid hormone is because of thyroid hormone resistance. Thyroid hormone resistance occurs when the thyroid receptor cells have an increased resistance to thyroid hormone, similar to many diabetic patients having an increased resistance to insulin. The end result is that these hypothyroid individuals may need more thyroid hormone to overcome this resistance. The blood tests do not recognize this increased resistance. Many conditions such as nutrient deficiencies are thought to block thyroid hormone at the cellular level, thus producing a clinically low thyroid state with normal blood indices. All too often, physicians rely on laboratory work to make their diagnosis, ignoring the patients' clinical condition, such as being fatigued or being cold, etc. A wise physician in medical school told me, "The patient will always tell you their diagnosis, if you will listen to them. You should never rely solely on the lab to make the diagnosis." I believe there would be a lot less untreated hypothyroidism if physicians heeded this advice today. Dr. Gerald Levy, an endocrinologist and chief of medicine at University of Pittsburgh School of Medicine, feels that there are many unknown factors that affect conventional testing including drugs and disease states. He feels hypothyroidism is a subtle disease that can easily be missed by conventional testing.[4]

Dr. Broda O. Barnes

Any discussion of the thyroid gland would be incomplete without giving credit to a great pioneer—Broda O. Barnes, M.D. Dr. Barnes wrote over 100 publications pertaining to the diagnosis and treatment of hypothyroidism. Through his exhaustive research, he determined that up to 40% of our population may be suffering needlessly from the ravages of hypothyroidism. How can one condition cause illness for up to 40% of our population? This number may sound far-fetched, but my experience reflects this high percentage and other practitioners who use natural hormones report similar findings. The Colorado Thyroid Disease Prevalence Study found that 10% of the population would have a thyroid abnormality based solely on blood tests.[5] When you factor in the clinical signs and symptoms, the numbers begin to approach Dr. Barnes' estimate.

Before the advent of antibiotics, Dr. Barnes' research illustrated that people with hypothyroidism often died before procreating. Adults who survived were those who were resistant to infection. He explains this in his book, _Hypothyroidism, the Unsuspected Illness_ (a book I highly recommend to all who are interested in promoting good health). Prior to the invention of antibiotics, the number one killer of children and young people was infection, primarily pneumonia. In fact, more than half of all children died of infections before reaching puberty. What did those people have that made them more susceptible to infections and died at such a young age? By reviewing over 70,000 autopsy reports, Dr. Barnes determined that this segment of the population probably suffered from hypothyroidism, which is known to make a person more susceptible to infection. Hypothyroidism can reduce the strength of every cell in the body, especially those responsible for maintaining the immune system.[6] As antibiotic use became more widespread, the population of hypothyroid people began surviving infections, living to an older age and procreating. Furthermore, these individuals began passing on their predisposition to hypothyroidism to the next generation and further generations to come.

This new population of hypothyroid people, now surviving infections and living to an older age, began exhibiting other signs of hypothyroidism, including atherosclerosis. After antibiotics were introduced in the 1940's, coronary artery disease (a consequence of hypothyroidism), quickly replaced infections as the number one killer in this country and remains the number one killer of adults today. It is my belief that many of the people suffering from atherosclerosis may have undiagnosed hypothyroidism.

Millions of dollars are spent in the United States on the treatment of the symptoms of coronary artery disease, including expensive and invasive procedures such as bypass surgery and balloon angioplasty. Many lives, as well as a tremendous amount of health care dollars, could be saved if we probed deeper and actually treated the cause of coronary artery disease rather than the symptoms. The cause of coronary artery disease is often blamed on high cholesterol levels. However, I believe it is not the high cholesterol that is the problem but, rather, untreated hypothyroidism that often is the root cause of high cholesterol levels and coronary artery disease. It has been known for decades that one of the consequences of hypothyroidism is elevated cholesterol levels and coronary artery disease. From my clinical experience, many people suffering from the ravages of coronary artery disease and elevated cholesterol levels can have their condition greatly improved when their hypothyroidism is appropriately diagnosed and treated.

James, a 58-year-old mechanic had been suffering from angina (i.e., chest pain) for eight years. He had a heart attack at age 49 and had been diagnosed with coronary artery disease. His cholesterol level averaged 260ng/dl (normal below 200ng/dl). James would use Nitroglycerin tablets, a prescription medication used to treat chest pain, approximately three times per week to control his angina. He had tried numerous cholesterol-lowering medications but could not tolerate their side effects. James had a basal temperature averaging 96.9 degrees Fahrenheit—fully one degree below normal. Upon taking Armour thyroid hormone, his angina symptoms resolved in a matter of weeks. Furthermore, his cholesterol level dropped to 195ng/dl. Three years later, James remains free of angina and reports, "I can now exercise without any chest pain. Before taking the thyroid hormone, I didn't have the energy to exercise and I would get chest pains at the start of any exercise. I can't believe how good I feel."

You might expect that over time, hypothyroid people would marry people with a normal functioning thyroid gland, thus decreasing the incidence of hypothyroidism. However, this isn't the case. Dr. Barnes wrote 20 years ago, "Experience has shown that more often than not, one thyroid-deficient person often marries another, helping to perpetuate and even increase the incidence of the trait."[7] I have observed similar findings in my practice. This idea makes sense if you consider that people will be attracted to others with the same energy level.

Joyce, 48-years-old, came to my office with complaints of feeling fatigued her whole life. She claimed, "My mother used to tell me I was born tired." She described a life of being constantly fatigued while trying to muster enough energy to just simply get through every day. She never had the strength to sustain any exercise program and complained of being constantly cold and having cold hands and feet. Joyce's basal temperature averaged 96.5 degrees Fahrenheit—over one degree lower than normal. She began taking Armour thyroid and reported, "I felt like I had awoken from a deep sleep." Now, she exercises daily and has begun an ambitious home improvement schedule. Chuck, Joyce's husband, could not keep up with her new activity level and she asked me to evaluate him as well. He also had a low basal temperature, and complained of being fatigued most of the time. He was started on Armour thyroid, which quickly restored his energy level to normal. Joyce recently reported, "We're doing more projects now than we did when we were first married. Now that Chuck is taking Armour thyroid, he is able to keep up with my schedule."

Environmental and dietary factors can also lead to hypothyroidism. My medical practice is situated in the center of the "goiter belt", which is named for the iodine-depleted soils in the Midwestern United States. Goiter belts are found throughout the world in inland regions where the soil and water are iodine depleted. In coastal areas, the soil and water contain adequate amounts of iodine. Iodine-depleted areas in the United States include the Great Lakes Basin and westward through Minnesota, South Dakota, North Dakota, Montana, Wyoming, the Rocky Mountains and into parts of the Northwest. In addition, many parts of Canada are found to have iodine-depleted areas.[8]

The thyroid gland is the main reservoir of iodine in the body. Iodine deficiency causes a goiter or swelling of the thyroid gland. According to Dr. Barnes, the replacement of iodine in our food supply, primarily through the use of iodized salt, has reduced the incidence of goiters but has not changed the incidence of hypothyroidism.[9] This may be due to environmental and hereditary factors inhibiting thyroid function as explained below.

Fluoride, which is added to most of the water supply in the United States, has been shown in numerous studies to inhibit thyroid function and possibly inhibit iodine uptake in the thyroid gland. Foods such as cabbage, cauliflower, kale, mustard greens, and turnips contain a compound called progoitrin, which can inhibit thyroid function. Walnuts, soy products, brussel sprouts, and millet can exacerbate thyroid problems.[10] In addition, radiation and chemotherapy can inhibit proper thyroid function. I have observed that almost all people who have received chemotherapy have thyroid abnormalities to some extent and most improve with the use of desiccated thyroid hormone such as Armour thyroid.

Environmental pollutants are also to blame. Phthalates, which are chemicals normally added to plastic, have been shown to cause hypothyroidism.[11] When you consider the amount of beverages consumed from plastic bottles in this country, the effects on the thyroid gland may be staggering. Due to the high incidence of thyroid and other hormonal disorders I see in my practice, I am convinced environmental pollutants play a significant role in causing thyroid and other hormonal imbalances in many people. Table 1 (page 44) shows other agents that may cause the thyroid gland to malfunction. For more information on how these agents cause the thyroid gland to malfunction, I refer the reader to my book, Overcoming Thyroid Disorders.

Dosage

Desiccated thyroid comes in pill form in varying strengths. This medication must be followed closely by a physician. It is imperative to follow serial blood tests and basal temperatures to find the optimum thyroid dose. Armour thyroid must initially be prescribed in low doses and titrated up to achieve the optimum result.

The best results with thyroid hormone are achieved when it is prescribed along with other natural hormones (e.g., DHEA, natural progesterone, etc.) to balance the entire hormonal system. This will be explained further in this book.

Side Effects

If desiccated thyroid (or any thyroid preparation) is taken in too large a dose, it can result in an over stimulation of the body, causing racing of the heart and palpitations. These symptoms, if untreated, can lead to serious health problems. A health care provider knowledgeable in the use of thyroid and other hormones should closely monitor thyroid hormone therapy.

Nutritional Support for the Thyroid Gland

Dietary recommendations for proper thyroid function include Vitamin A- 5,000I.U., Vitamin B3- 1,000mg, Vitamin B6- 100mg, Vitamin B Complex 100mg, Vitamin B12- 1,000mcg, Vitamin C- 3,000mg, Vitamin E- 400 IU and Selenium- 200mcg daily. Also, 64 oz. of pure water per day (fluoride-free) as well as foods high in iodine, such as seafood, are helpful for promoting a healthy thyroid. I have found that nutritional supplements, although helpful, do not generally improve thyroid function as efficiently as combining them with small amounts of desiccated thyroid hormone, when indicated.

Final Thoughts

It is very difficult for the body to convert inactive thyroid hormone to active thyroid hormone without adequate iron stores available. It is imperative to be checked for anemia before beginning any thyroid hormone replacement therapy. I recommend checking a serum ferritin level, which is a measure of iron stores in the body, before treating with thyroid hormone. Low iron levels are easily treated with iron supplementation.

Adequate thyroid production is necessary for the proper functioning of every other endocrine gland in the body, including the adrenal glands. Insufficient thyroid hormone production will lead to a dysfunctional hormonal system. My experience has shown that it is impossible to balance the other endocrine glands in the body without first addressing a thyroid imbalance.

It is imperative to keep in mind the interrelationships of all of the hormones in the body. When I prescribe natural hormones, I generally prescribe them in combinations. Using combinations of natural hormones is more effective than using the hormones individually. My clinical experience has shown that combinations of natural hormones have a synergistic effect with one another. The following Chapters will illustrate this point.

[1] Richman, J., et al. A community based study of chronic fatigue syndrome. Arch. Int. Med. 1999;159(18):2129

[2] Lindstedt, Goran. Thyroid dysfunction and chronic fatigue. Letter. Lancet. Vol. 358. July, 2001

[3] Barnes, Broda. Hypothyroidism, The Unsuspected Illness. Harper and Row. 1976

[4] Hypothyroidism, a treacherous masquerader. Acute Care Medicine, May, 1984.

[5] Archives of Int. Medicine. Vol. 150, No. 4. 2/28/2000

[6] IBID. Barnes, Broda.

[7] IBID. Barnes, Broda.

[8] Langer, Stephen. Solved: The Riddle of Illness. Keats, p. 18, 1995

[9] IBID. Barnes, Broda.

[10] IBID. Langer, Stephen.

[11] IBID. Langer, Stephen.

Chapter 4

Adrenal Hormones Introduction

Introduction

The adrenal glands sit at the top of the kidneys in the back. The adrenal glands are broken down into two sections: the adrenal medulla and the adrenal cortex.

The adrenal medulla produces the "flight or fight" hormones that prepare the body for stress. These include the adrenal hormones epinephrine and nor-epinephrine.

The adrenal cortex produces steroid hormones that serve multiple functions including helping the body to fight infections, heal from injuries and regulate blood sugar metabolism. The main type of hormone produced in the adrenal cortex is hydrocortisone. Hydrocortisone provides the body with glucose and amino acids necessary for the body's metabolism, especially in stressful states.

Sex hormones are also produced in the adrenal cortex (as well as in the ovaries and the testicles). These hormones include the androgen (i.e., tissue and muscle building) hormones pregnenolone, DHEA, and testosterone. DHEA and testosterone are responsible for building muscles and healing injured areas of the body.

Progesterone and estrogens are also produced in the adrenal glands in men and women. In women, progesterone and estrogen are primarily produced in the ovaries until menopause when the adrenal glands become the primary endocrine source for estrogen production. In men, the adrenal cortex serves as one of the primary sources for the production of progesterone and estrogen.

Life is incompatible without adrenal hormones. Adrenal hormones help the body adapt to changes (i.e., stressors) in the environment. An imbalance in the production and secretion of the adrenal hormones can often manifest as illness. I have found that it is vitally important to check hormone levels for proper adrenal gland functioning and provide the necessary natural hormones to help the body in times of illness.

My experience has shown that the most common problem associated with the adrenal glands is adrenal insufficiency, or low adrenal hormone output. The next few chapters will illustrate the beneficial effects of using natural adrenal hormones to restore balance to the body.

There is a close interaction between the adrenal glands and the thyroid gland. If there is inadequate production in one gland there will be serious consequences for the other gland. For example, if hypothyroidism is present, adrenal imbalances will often be found. My clinical experience has repeatedly shown that the best results are obtained by properly balancing both systems simultaneously with the use of combinations of natural hormones.

Figure 4 illustrates the production of the adrenal hormones. Note that all of the adrenal hormones are produced from the fat-like substance cholesterol. Chapters 5-12 will discuss each hormone individually.

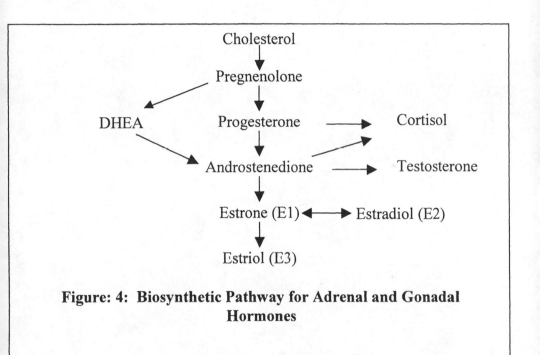

Figure: 4: Biosynthetic Pathway for Adrenal and Gonadal Hormones

Chapter 5

DHEA

BENEFITS OF DHEA

The benefits of taking DHEA include preventing and treating: Alzheimer's, asthma and allergies, bacterial and viral infections, cancer, cardiovascular disease, diabetes, hypertension, high cholesterol, obesity, osteoporosis and immune system diseases including AIDS. I have also found DHEA particularly effective for treating autoimmune disorders such as fibromyalgia, rheumatoid arthritis, lupus, Crohn's, and others.

Introduction

DHEA is an acronym for dehydroepiandrosterone, an androgen hormone produced in the adrenal glands. The adrenal glands are found adjacent to the kidneys and are necessary for the production of many different hormones such as DHEA, progesterone, estrogen, testosterone, pregnenolone, and cortisone. DHEA is the most abundant steroid produced in the body and DHEA sulfate is the most abundant form of DHEA. (The other hormones mentioned above will be covered in future chapters.) DHEA is secreted into the blood stream and is converted by the liver to DHEA sulfate (DHEA-S). All DHEA levels mentioned in this book are the DHEA-S form. DHEA should only be measured in the sulfate form, DHEA-S.

The adrenal glands are responsible for the body's hormonal response to stress—the "fight or flight" reaction. When the body is placed under a stressful situation, the adrenal glands respond by increasing the output of their hormones, including DHEA. This increased production is necessary to help the body adjust to any stressful situation such as infection, injury or illness. When the adrenal glands malfunction and decrease the production of their hormones, the body's capacity to withstand disease and promote healing becomes compromised. In fact, in severe disease states, DHEA and other adrenal hormones are known to have severely depressed levels. I have observed that physiologic doses of DHEA and other natural hormones are essential in treating these severe disease states. In addition, I have observed that it is necessary to maintain DHEA levels near their peak in order to achieve the best results, as explained in the Discussion section. The peak DHEA levels for women range from 1,200-3,000ng/ml and the peak DHEA levels for men range from 2,000-4,000ng/ml (see page 76).

Case Studies

Headaches

Marsha is 30 years old and has suffered from headaches for 15 years. Marsha reported having a headache virtually every day of her life. Associated with her daily headaches are occasional migraine headaches. Marsha tried numerous prescription medications without relief. "I don't really know what it is like to go through a whole day without a headache," she stated. She also complained, "I get every cold that comes around. I am constantly sick. My immune system cannot be functioning

well. My friends at work cannot believe how often I get sick."
Marsha had a basal temperature that averaged 97.8 degrees
Fahrenheit. In Chapter 3 we established that he normal basal
temperature ranges from 97.8-98.2 degrees Fahrenheit. Marsha's
DHEA level was low at 950ng/ml. She was placed on 10mg of
DHEA per day and reported marked improvement in her
symptoms. Within three weeks, her headaches were markedly
decreased. Furthermore, her DHEA level improved to a healthy
2,900ng/ml. Marsha also stopped getting every viral and bacterial
illness that was going around. "I can't believe how much better I
feel. My headaches are almost totally gone and I am not getting
sick all the time," she commented.

Marsha's case illustrates how each of us is unique. Thyroid
hormone may be lacking in one person with headaches, as seen in
Chapter 3, while DHEA may be lacking in others with headaches.
I believe over 75% of people who suffer from chronic headaches,
including migraine headaches, have a hormonal imbalance.

Dayna, a 17-year-old high school student, suffered from
migraine headaches. Her headaches began at age 12. Dayna said,
"When I get a migraine, my head feels like it is going to explode. I
cannot stand any light and I get very nauseous. I can't do
anything but lie in bed until it passes, usually for two to three
days." Her headaches occurred approximately two times per
week. Dayna became so debilitated from her headaches that she
had basically dropped out of high school. Dayna had tried
numerous prescription medicines that either did nothing or had

side effects that made her feel worse. She had been admitted to a hospital to try various treatments, but none of them helped. Dayna reported her headaches worsened during allergy season, usually in the fall. She used to love riding horses, but had to give this up claiming that "riding on the horse made my headaches worse." Dayna's DHEA level was only 900ng/ml. When Dayna started taking 5mg of DHEA per day, she noticed an improvement within two weeks. The frequency and intensity of her migraines began declining. At a two-month check-up she reported feeling 95% better and commented, "It feels like a miracle, my headaches are gone. I haven't had one in over four weeks. The best thing is I've started riding my horse again. In fact, now I ride every day. I haven't been able to ride my horse for almost five years because of the persistent headaches." She also reported a significant increase in her energy level. "I didn't realize how tired I was all the time," she said.

Headaches have multifactorial cause. Headaches that start around the time of menarche (i.e., the beginning of a menstrual period), or headaches that repeatedly occur during the same time of the menstrual cycle are usually a sign of a hormonal imbalance and generally respond favorably to natural hormonal therapies, as in Dayna's case.

Allergies and Asthma

David, a 36-year- old physician, suffered with asthma and allergies since he was five years old. He was treated with numerous allergy and asthma medications that caused many side effects. "I was constantly drowsy from the medications and I was always using inhalers. They helped a little bit, but I would wheeze most nights from spring until winter," he said. David's DHEA level was very low at 850ng/ml. David was told to drink more water for a dehydrated condition (see Chapter 13) and take 5mg of DHEA per day. When David started taking the DHEA, he noticed an immediate change in his symptoms. "My asthma symptoms improved dramatically. About 80% of my allergy and asthma symptoms went away with the DHEA. I now take no allergy medications and I only use the inhalers when I exercise strenuously. I feel like a new person," he happily commented.

David is your author. DHEA supplementation has made a remarkable improvement in my allergy and asthma symptoms. Since improving, I have treated many patients for asthma and allergy symptoms with DHEA and noticed similar improvements. Dr. William Jeffries, an endocrinologist at Case Western Reserve, has observed that many patients with allergies have evidence of low adrenal function and will improve with physiologic supplementation of adrenal hormones.[1] My experience has indicated that all allergy and asthma sufferers should be examined for a hormonal imbalance and should supplement with DHEA (as well as other natural hormones) when indicated.

Cheryl, a 32-year-old homemaker, had a five-year history of multiple allergies to food and environmental agents. She was well until she had a viral infection five years ago. "I've just never recovered from that cold," she stated. Since that time, she complained of constant headaches, loss of energy, and constant nasal congestion with drainage. Cheryl was very athletic but could no longer exercise due to her fatigue. She had been treated with numerous antibiotics for sinusitis that would help her congestion temporarily. Her initial DHEA level was 850ng/ml. She started taking 10mg of DHEA per day, and reported improvement in her symptoms almost immediately. In addition, she noticed that her energy level improved and that she was able to exercise again. Her DHEA level improved to a healthy 2,800ng/ml. Many allergic people will have a suppressed DHEA level, and will find that their symptoms improve with DHEA supplementation.

Ulcerative Colitis

Mark, a 44-year-old typesetter, had a two-year history of ulcerative colitis, an autoimmune disease causing bleeding of the colon. His gastroenterologist believed a colectomy (i.e., removal of the colon) was necessary to control his symptoms. Prednisone is a synthetic steroid hormone often prescribed for this condition, but it has many harmful side effects. Mark did not want a colectomy and he came to me for a second opinion. Mark's original DHEA level was 890ng/ml. After taking 30mg of DHEA per day, his level elevated to 4072ng/ml and he felt much better. His bloody diarrhea gradually resolved over two months and he has been symptom free for four years.

In my practice, I have found that close to 100% of patients with autoimmune diseases such as Crohn's, ulcerative colitis, lupus, multiple sclerosis, rheumatoid arthritis, fibromyalgia and others have significantly depressed DHEA levels. In addition, most of these patients show clinical improvement in their condition upon using physiologic replacement doses of DHEA. A study on patients suffering from severe lupus was conducted at Stanford University and it showed that DHEA supplementation improved the patients' disease states as well as reduced their need for high dose steroids.[2] Are these chronic diseases a function of low DHEA levels or vice versa? I do not have the answer, but my clinical observation is that people with chronic diseases will have their condition significantly improved with DHEA supplementation, when it is indicated.

Hypertension

Dennis, a 52-year-old CEO of a manufacturing company had been using antihypertensive medications for 10 years. He was being treated with Procardia, an antihypertensive drug, to help lower his blood pressure. Dennis complained of having aching joints and muscles. He was found to be hypothyroid and was treated with Armour thyroid hormone. "With the Armour thyroid, I feel so much better. My achiness is 80% better," he said. However, Dennis' blood pressure failed to lower with the thyroid medication. Dennis had a DHEA level of 880ng/ml. Upon taking 20mg of DHEA, all of his remaining muscle aches cleared-- almost overnight. In addition, he was able to stop taking his antihypertensive medication, and still maintain a normal blood pressure. Dennis was ecstatic and commented, "All of my achiness is gone. I don't lift weights, but I feel stronger and my muscles, which were slowly deteriorating as I aged, have started to come back. I feel as good as I've ever felt. Also, I'm glad I don't have to take that blood pressure medicine, I have never felt right on it. The best part is that I am hitting the golf ball better than ever."

Dennis received the most improvement from his symptoms when the Armour thyroid hormone was taken in conjunction with DHEA, again pointing toward a synergistic effect with using combinations of hormones. I have often found hypertension responds favorably to DHEA and other natural hormonal support. In most hypertensive cases, my patients are able to significantly reduce or eliminate prescription medications when they are treated with natural hormones.

Cancer

Cancer patients, especially those with metastatic disease, have very suppressed DHEA levels. There is some controversy about using DHEA with hormone-sensitive cancers such as breast or prostate cancer. There is concern that DHEA may worsen the course of hormone-sensitive cancer. If you suffer from breast or prostate cancer, the use of DHEA must be discussed with your doctor. I have treated a number of cancer patients—all with approval from their oncologist—with DHEA and almost all of them experienced dramatic clinical improvements in their condition. Cancer patients generally report feeling markedly better and having higher energy levels when supplemented with DHEA (when indicated). In addition, their laboratory values improve and they appear to have a less active disease. Also, DHEA helps cancer patients tolerate chemotherapy with less adverse symptoms. Due to my positive experience using DHEA, I predict DHEA supplementation, with its effects on improving the function of the immune system, will be a priority for most cancer patients in the future.

Emily, a 46-year-old homemaker and mother of three, was diagnosed with breast cancer two years ago. Since undergoing surgery and radiation, she has never felt the same. Emily lamented, "I have lost my energy. I used to be a vibrant, active person who could work from the moment I got up until late at night. Now, I can barely get anything done during the day because I'm so tired. I feel like I've aged 20 years since my treatment." Emily's DHEA level was low at 295ng/ml. Upon taking 10mg of DHEA per day, Emily noticed an immediate improvement in her condition. "Two days after starting DHEA, I felt like I was waking up," she said. After six weeks, she reported, "I am beginning to feel like my old self. My energy level feels like it has been jump-started." At a six-month check-up, Emily reported that she had regained all of her energy. Her DHEA level improved to 2,600ng/ml. Emily has since started a vigorous exercise program and has spoken at her church about the benefits of natural therapies.

Fibromyalgia

I have found a correlation between low DHEA levels and

fibromyalgia, a painful condition characterized by aching of the muscles and fatigue. There is no known cause of or cure for fibromyalgia. I have seen many fibromyalgia patients improve through the use of natural hormones.

Ruth, 46 years old, had complained for years of pains in her back and her arms. Ruth had seen neurologists and orthopedic surgeons who told her she had fibromyalgia. They tried injecting trigger points and giving her non-steroidal anti-inflammatory medications, all without relief. Ruth's condition gradually worsened to the point that she began dropping objects. Ruth said, "I feel like an old person. I have occasionally dropped a drinking glass because it feels too heavy for my arms. Besides dropping things, I can't stand to be in pain every day." Ruth was found to have an initial DHEA level of 820ng/ml. Her DHEA level rapidly improved to 2,800ng/ml upon taking 20mg of DHEA per day. More importantly, her pain almost completely resolved within two weeks of starting the DHEA. Ruth claimed, "It truly feels like a miracle. I think I started to feel better the next day after starting the DHEA. Within one week, I noticed my pain was totally gone. I used to be very sore after golfing, but now I feel great when I am done."

Discussion

The adrenal glands produce their hormones in a sequential order. DHEA is often referred to as a "precursor hormone" because DHEA is converted in the body to other hormones such as testosterone and estrogen. DHEA may be able to raise progesterone levels as well. Since DHEA is so integral to the production of these other hormones, if DHEA production is suppressed, the production of testosterone, estrogen and progesterone is likewise suppressed. This decreased production of hormones can be manifested as an increased susceptibility to illness as well as an acceleration of the aging process.

DHEA levels peak around 20-30 years of age and gradually decline as we get older (see Figure 5). Are these declining DHEA levels a mechanism for triggering the aging process? I do not have the answer, but I have found that increasing the level of DHEA to its peak level is beneficial in treating illness as well as slowing down the signs of aging. The Baltimore Longitudinal Study of Aging showed that men who had higher DHEA-S levels had significantly greater longevity as compared to men with lower levels.[3] An Italian study showed a direct relationship between DHEA levels and functional independence in people over 90 years old.[4]

Supplementation with DHEA has also been shown to help prevent depression and improve mood in individuals with low DHEA levels.[5] [6] Positive psychological changes with DHEA supplementation (including enhancements in self-esteem and mood and a decrease in fatigue) have also been shown in a more recent study.[7] In women, low DHEA levels were found to be significantly associated with depression, regardless of the age.[8]

Most people respond positively to DHEA supplementation (when indicated). A study at the University of California showed that using physiologic doses of DHEA was associated with a remarkable increase in physical and psychological well-being for the majority of men and women in the study.[9]

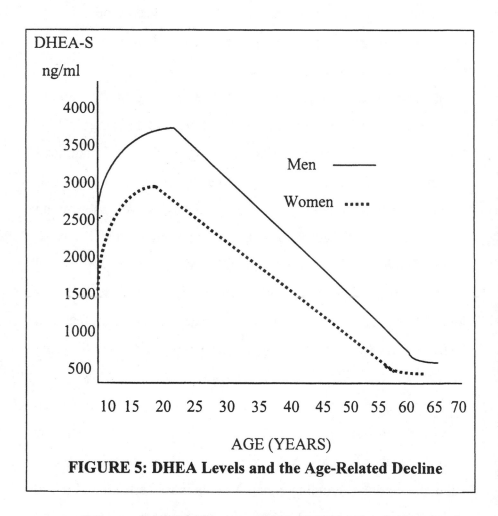

FIGURE 5: DHEA Levels and the Age-Related Decline

I have observed consistently low DHEA levels in elderly patients as well as most individuals suffering from any chronic disease condition such as lupus, Crohn's, ulcerative colitis, fibromyalgia, diabetes, multiple sclerosis, etc. In prolonged stressful states, such as chronic illness, Dr. Jeffries has shown how the adrenal glands may underfunction by producing subnormal levels of DHEA and other adrenal hormones. He has published numerous articles and books describing the benefits of using physiologic doses of adrenal hormones to address the various chronic conditions mentioned above.[10] It is well known that individuals with chronic conditions often appear to age quickly and have many clinical signs of advanced aging. DHEA supplementation can produce noticeable improvements in aging parameters including less muscle wasting and wrinkling of the skin, less fatigue and improved muscle mass. Dr. Alan Gaby, a well-known researcher on the use of natural treatments, has observed similar results,[11] as have most of my colleagues who have experience with prescribing DHEA

DHEA also possesses anti-cancer properties. In rats predisposed to getting prostate cancer, DHEA conferred significant protection against prostate cancer.[12 13]

DHEA is presently found over-the-counter at health food stores and I have even seen it at grocery stores. People taking this hormone need to know it is a powerful hormonal compound and should not be taken lightly. This is not like taking something relatively innocuous like Vitamin C. Though I discuss the benefits of DHEA, I want to emphasize that it should only be taken under monitored conditions. DHEA levels should be checked and the health care professional recommending its usage should be knowledgeable and have experience with prescribing DHEA. When it is used appropriately, DHEA is very safe. I feel in the near future we are going to see negative side effects of DHEA as a result of people taking excessive doses without the proper guidance from a health care practitioner. DHEA levels should be measured before and after supplementation with DHEA. In obtaining DHEA levels from various medical labs, normal ranges often vary between the different laboratories. I have found that adequate levels for men range from 2,000-4,000ng/dl and for women from 1,200-3,000ng/dl. These levels closely approximate the peak levels of DHEA seen in Figure 5 and have been found to be safe. In treating chronic illness, I have often found it necessary to raise DHEA levels to approximate the peak levels mentioned above.

Dosage

Natural DHEA is produced from plant products and has the same chemical structure as DHEA produced in the human body. The dosage of DHEA varies between persons and depends on their condition. Generally, the more severely ill a person is, the more DHEA will be required to bring their level into a normal range. Patients with an autoimmune disease or cancer will generally need more DHEA than other patients. DHEA should be taken on an empty stomach for better absorption. DHEA should not be compounded with lactose, which is used as a filler. Lactose may cause stomach upset. Either olive oil or ginger is a better choice for the filler. I have found the use of small doses of DHEA, in the range of 2-5mg/day for women and 5-10mg per day for men, are effective in treating the majority of patients.

Side Effects

Side effects of using physiologic doses of DHEA are rare. The side effects I have witnessed have been acne and moodiness occurring in approximately 5% of my patients, usually young females. I have also noticed mild hair growth occurring in 1% of my patients, which is easily managed with a dose reduction.

Nutritional Support for the Adrenal Glands

Dietary recommendations for the adrenal glands include: Vitamin C-3,000mg/day (one of the highest concentrations of Vitamin C is in the adrenal glands), Vitamin A-5,000mg/day, Vitamin E-400IU/day and Pantothenic Acid-500mg/day. Dietary factors include drinking adequate amounts of pure water per day and having adequate salt intake using unrefined Celtic Sea Salt. Herbal therapies can include licorice root 600mg/day and Gotu Kola 50-100mg/day. Adrenal glandulars have also been very helpful for many different conditions. The best results with DHEA have occurred when DHEA is combined with the appropriate nutritional supplementation.

A Word Of Caution

When I go into a health food store and see many jars of DHEA on the shelves, I am concerned about the high doses readily available without proper monitoring of levels. I rarely use doses greater than 10mg per day. Large doses that are not indicated may cause problems with adrenal gland suppression.

Final Thoughts

There are many drugs that may negatively impact DHEA production. These can include many of the hypertensive drugs, including calcium channel blockers, beta-blockers and others. I have found hypertension can often be improved with supplementation of DHEA. The first step to treating an illness, such as hypertension, is to give the body substances (like DHEA) that will help improve the functioning of the immune and hormonal systems.

[1] Mck. Jeffries, William. Safe Uses of Cortisol. Thomas, 1996, p. 105
[2] Van Vollenhovenm, Ronald. Arthritis and Rheumatism, September, 1994;37Z(9);1305-10
[3] Science 2002. Aug. 2, 297 (5582):811
[4] Ravaglia, G., et al. The relationship of dehydroepiandrosterone sulfate (DHEAS) to endocrine-metabolic parameters and functional status in the oldest-old. Results from an Italian study on healthy free-living over-,inety-year olds. J. Clin. Endocrin. Metab. 1996;81(3):1173-8
[5] Wolkowitz, O.M., et al. Dehydroepiandrosterone (DHEA) treatment of depression. Biol. Psychiatry. 1997. Feb. 1;41(3):311-8
[6] Wolkowita, O.M., et al. Double-blind treatment of major depression with dehydroepiandrosterone. Am.J. Psychiatry. 1999. Apr;156(4):646-9
[7] Hunt, P, et al. Improvement in mood and fatigue after dehydroepiandrosterone replacement in Addison's disease in a randomized, double blind trial. J. Clin.Ednocrin. Metab. 2000;85(12);4650-6
[8] Barrett-Conner, E., et al. Endogenous levels of dehydroepiandrosterone sulfate, but not other hormones, are associated with depressed mood in older women: Rancho Bernardo Study. Am. Geriatr. Soc. 1999. Jun;47(6):685-91
[9] Morales, Arlene, et al. Effects of replacement dose of dehydroepiandrosterone in men and women of advancing age. Journal of Clinical Endocrinology and Metabolism. 1994;78;1360-67
[10] Mck. Jeffries, William. IBID. 1976
[11] Gaby, Alan. Holistic Medicine. Spring, 1995
[12] Rao, KV, ct al. Chcmoprcvention of rat prostate carcinogenesis by early and delayed administration of dehydroepiandrosterone. Cancer Res. 1999, Jul 1;59(13)3084-9
[13] McCormick, DL, et al. Chemoprevention of hormone-dependant prostate cacner in the Wistar-Unilever rat. Eur. Urol. 1999;35 (5-6):464-7

Chapter 6

Progesterone

Introduction

Progesterone is one of two main hormones produced by the ovaries. The other main ovarian hormone is estrogen. Progesterone is primarily produced in the second half of the woman's menstrual cycle and is the hormone necessary for the survival of the fetus. Men produce very tiny amounts of progesterone from the testicles. In men and women, a small amount of progesterone is also produced in the adrenal glands, where it acts as a precursor for the adrenal estrogens, testosterone, and cortical steroids, described in later chapters. There are two types of progesterone currently available: natural progesterone and synthetic progesterone (e.g., Provera). Natural progesterone is made from plant products and has the same chemical structure as the progesterone that is produced in the human body. The difference in the chemical structures of natural progesterone and Provera are illustrated in Figure 7, page 97. I have found natural progesterone safer and much more effective for treating illness and promoting health than synthetic progesterone. This will be explained more fully in the Case Studies and the Discussion sections.

Case Studies

PMS and Menstrual Irregularities

Betty, a 48-year-old beautician, complained of increased bleeding with her menses as well as worsening PMS symptoms. She had tried Provera, a synthetic progesterone, but reported, "It only made my symptoms worse." Betty's progesterone level on day 21 of her cycle was 8ng/ml (normal progesterone level is 20-30ng/ml). After starting natural progesterone, she noticed an improvement right away. "My family is so happy my moods have improved, they want to take you out to dinner," she told me two months later. Her progesterone level improved to a healthy 24ng/ml. Later, Betty went to her gynecologist for a pap smear and was told natural progesterone was "garbage" and that she should throw it out. When she tried to explain to the doctor how much better she felt, he would not listen. When I called the doctor to discuss this, I asked him how much experience he had with natural progesterone. He answered "None." Needless to say, Betty elected to stay on natural progesterone and asked me to recommend a new gynecologist.

Unfortunately, most doctors are unaware of the therapeutic value of natural hormones, and therefore are quite skeptical of their benefits. My response to this skepticism is based on the symptom relief my patients have had upon using natural hormones, after having failed to improve with other treatments. Furthermore, as the Women's Health Study Initiative showed (see Chapter 2), there is no indication for using a synthetic hormone, when a natural hormone is available.

Brenda, at 32 years old, was suffering from severe PMS. She complained that her husband was threatening to leave her. She said, "I wouldn't blame him if he did. I have two weeks out of the month when I feel human, and two weeks out of the month where I turn into this moody, nasty person. My co-workers know to stay away from me during this time. I really do feel sorry for my husband, but I can't control it." In addition, she was having very heavy menstrual periods. "It feels like I am hemorrhaging every time I have a period," she said. Brenda's doctor prescribed birth control pills, which did help with some of her PMS symptoms, but she began getting headaches and noticing fatigue. Brenda's progesterone level on Day 21 of her cycle was 12ng/ml, about half of what it should be. Upon taking natural progesterone, Brenda's PMS gradually resolved over three months. Furthermore, the heavy bleeding during her periods ceased. A recent laboratory test showed that her progesterone level was elevated to 24ng/ml on day 21 of her cycle. "I can't believe this is how a normal period should feel,' she said. Brenda now reports having minimal discomfort and a manageable amount of bleeding during her menses.

Danielle, 38 years old, complained of extremely heavy menstrual bleeding. She claimed, "I have to take a day off work every month because the bleeding and cramping are so severe." Furthermore, she complained of feeling fatigued and having severe PMS symptoms including mood swings, headaches and depression for up to five days before her period. Danielle's progesterone level on day 21 of her cycle was 8.6ng/ml (normal 20-30ng/ml). Danielle was drinking three cups of coffee every day and craving chocolate at the end of her cycle. Caffeine intake has been shown in numerous studies to be related to PMS symptoms.[1] Therefore, the first step to Danielle's treatment plan was to have her eliminate caffeine including chocolate, which contains caffeine. Next, Danielle was placed on natural progesterone from days 14-28 of her cycle which closely mimics the body's own production cycle for progesterone. Danielle experienced a marked improvement in her mood swings, headaches, fatigue, and depression. In addition, her progesterone level improved to 27ng/ml. "Now I know what a normal period should feel like. I believe I have been given a new lease on life. I no longer feel like I am hemorrhaging every cycle and my bleeding is much more manageable. I can't believe I had to suffer for so many years when there was a natural treatment available," she stated.

Depression

Ellen, a 34-year-old homemaker, complained of having recurrent episodes of depression since her teenage years. Ellen had seen numerous doctors with her complaints. She said, "Doctors would not listen to me or take me seriously. They kept telling me I had PMS, but they could not offer me any relief. I began to think it was normal to suffer severe emotional swings and depression for 10-14 days before my period began. I tried birth control pills, which only made my symptoms worse. I have gotten to the point where I dread the two weeks before my period because I feel so terrible." Ellen also suffered from heavy menstrual bleeding and periodic episodes of hair loss. Ellen had a healthy lifestyle including drinking eight glasses of water per day and not ingesting any caffeine. "My healthy lifestyle made no difference in my symptoms," she said. Ellen had a progesterone level of 9.9ng/ml on day 21 of her menstrual cycle. Upon taking natural progesterone, her progesterone level improved to a healthy 26ng/ml. More importantly, all of her symptoms improved. Two-months after starting natural progesterone therapy Ellen reported, "I definitely feel better. I feel like I can handle life now. My PMS is totally gone and I'm not depressed. My energy has risen to a *level I don't ever remember having. I can't imagine feeling any better. I wish I had taken natural progesterone years ago so I wouldn't have suffered through all the depression. I now find that I can accomplish so much more during the month because I feel so much better. It is wonderful to have the mood swings gone and now I don't dread the two weeks before my period."*

Fibroid Tumors and Hypothyroidism

Susan, age 41, has been on Synthroid, a synthetic thyroid hormone for 15 years. For the last five years, she has noticed increasing PMS, heavy menstrual bleeding and the growth of fibroid tumors. Upon taking natural progesterone, her PMS and heavy menstrual bleeding immediately resolved. In addition, her fibroid tumors stopped increasing in size, thus averting a possible hysterectomy. I was also able to cut her Synthroid dose in half due to the beneficial effects natural progesterone has on thyroid hormone function. Natural progesterone makes thyroid hormone receptors more receptive to thyroid hormone (see Chapter 3 for more information).

Fibroid tumors are benign growths in the uterine muscular wall and are usually associated with pain and heavy bleeding. Fibroid tumors are thought to be a product of excess estrogen stimulation to the uterus. Besides a woman's own production of estrogen, environmental estrogen-like compounds are found in pesticides, petrochemicals and other pollution. This results in an excess estrogen stimulation in all of our bodies. Natural progesterone can counteract the excess estrogen stimulation that occurs in the body. When natural progesterone is used in a woman with fibroid tumors, the fibroid tumors will most likely stop enlarging and, many times will regress in size. It still amazes me that gynecologists will take a "wait and see" approach with fibroids until they are too large, thus necessitating surgery. There is a safe, natural treatment already available—natural progesterone.

Osteoporosis

Joyce, 63 years old was concerned about osteoporosis. "My mother was crippled by osteoporosis. I don't want to end up like her," she said. Joyce had a recent bone scan that showed that her bone density was declining, putting her at risk for osteoporosis. Joyce was prescribed drugs (Fosomax) to treat osteoporosis, but could not tolerate them. "The drugs made me very sick. I don't want osteoporosis, but I know I cannot take the drugs," she claimed. When I evaluated Joyce, I found very low progesterone and DHEA levels. Joyce was put on a program that included diet changes (reduction of refined foods), exercise, and natural hormonal therapies including natural progesterone and DHEA, along with vitamin and mineral supplements. Over the next three bone density tests, Joyce's bone density reversed itself. "My internist was amazed. He kept saying, "I have never seen this happen". I feel so much stronger on the natural hormones that I know I will not be bothered by osteoporosis," she claimed.

Many conventional physicians are under the mistaken belief that estrogens alone-- and synthetic estrogens at that-- are the best treatment for osteoporosis. However, they are ignoring the research. None of the studies show estrogen alone increases bone mass. Estrogen supplementation has only been shown to retard the progression of osteoporosis. Researchers have found progesterone receptors in cells specifically designed for bone building.[2] Due to overwhelming evidence of excess estrogen-like compounds in the environment and the fact that estrogen is continually produced in the postmenopausal woman, I frequently use natural progesterone without estrogen to combat osteoporosis. Studies have shown progesterone is able to increase bone mass in women, while estrogens can only retard the rate of bone loss. Dr. John Lee, author of *Natural Progesterone: The Multiple Roles of a Remarkable Hormone* writes, "I have treated postmenopausal osteoporosis with transdermal natural progesterone included in a program of diet, mineral and vitamin supplements, and modest exercise, and demonstrated true reversal of osteoporosis even in patients who did not use estrogen supplements."[3] I have also experienced similar findings in my patients.

Dr. Lee studied 63 patients measuring bone mineral density, which is a common measurement to gauge the degree of osteoporosis. He compared the bone mineral density of patients using natural progesterone, patients using estrogen and those using no hormonal therapies. Only the natural progesterone group showed an increase in bone mineral density, with the estrogen group maintaining bone density and the control group losing an average of 1.5% per year. Dr. Lee determined that lack of exercise, poor nutrition and progesterone deficiency are the major factors for causing osteoporosis.[4] Osteoporosis is a multifactorial problem and I refer the reader to a book by Dr. Alan Gaby, *Preventing and Reversing Osteoporosis.*

Discussion

In a menstruating woman, the ovaries and the adrenal glands produce progesterone. Figure 6 depicts the normal cycling of progesterone and estrogen during the menstrual cycle. In a typical 28-day cycle, progesterone levels start to rise about day 14. Progesterone levels rise during the second half of the cycle in anticipation of a possible fertilized ovum. If no implantation is made, menses begins around day 28 and a new cycle begins. In a post-menopausal woman, progesterone continues to be produced by the ovaries and the adrenal glands in smaller amounts as compared to the menstruating woman.

Estrogen is also produced by the ovaries in a cyclic fashion. Estrogen levels peak in the first part of the menstrual cycle and also peak in the second half of the cycle. In post-menopausal women, the ovaries produce smaller amounts of estrogen. Estrogen will be more thoroughly covered in the next chapter. A normal menstrual cycle is necessary for health. When the menstrual cycle is not functioning correctly, it sets the stage for disease states to occur, and it accelerates aging.

I define a normal menstrual cycle as having the following four characteristics:

1. The cycle occurs monthly.
2. The cycle contains the normal rise and fall of estrogen and progesterone, including ovulation.
3. The menstrual period should not be preceded by mood swings and discomfort—the stereotypical premenstrual syndrome (PMS).
4. There should be an average amount of bleeding and a minimal amount of discomfort while menstruating.

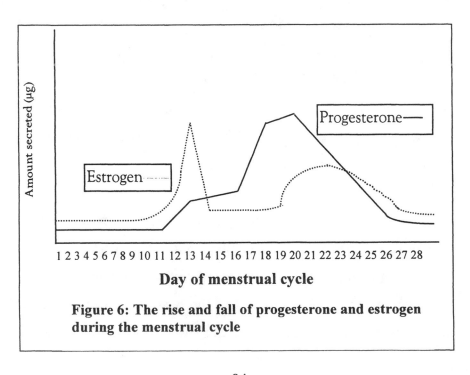

Figure 6: The rise and fall of progesterone and estrogen during the menstrual cycle

I have found with the proper use of natural hormones, most women will achieve this ideal cycle. When a menstrual cycle does not contain all of the above characteristics, there is most likely a hormonal problem. Frequently the problem is due to a progesterone deficiency.

Birth Control Pills

When a woman takes birth control pills, the normal menstrual cycle is inhibited and production of the body's own hormones are decreased. The beneficial effects of the woman's natural hormones, especially progesterone and estrogen, are inhibited. This loss of normal hormonal function does not promote health, and I believe it sets the stage for disease and aging to progress at an accelerated rate. Furthermore, birth control pills inhibit the proper function of other hormones including thyroid, DHEA and testosterone. These hormones are tissue building hormones. How can you expect the body to heal injured tissues if there is inhibition of natural hormonal production present?

Researchers found women taking birth control pills had a significant decrease of serum testosterone and DHEA levels.[5] I have observed in my practice that women who take birth control pills often have multiple hormonal imbalances. These hormonal imbalances usually improve when birth control pills are stopped. Furthermore, I have found that birth control pills can exacerbate and accelerate many chronic conditions, particularly autoimmune disorders.

Menopausal symptoms and osteoporosis are major concerns for post-menopausal women. If menopause and subsequent reduction of hormone production is a natural event, it may seem counter-intuitive for women to supplement with hormones. However, it is well known that women are more prone to disease and illness, including coronary artery disease and osteoporosis, after menopause. Through the use of natural hormones such as natural progesterone, I believe women can slow down and often reverse these disease processes and slow down many other signs of aging (e.g., wrinkling of the skin, wasting of the muscles). John Lee, M.D., states, "I don't think nature is to blame. Many plants contain progesterone and natural estrogens that help maintain health in people who consume them. In modern America we tend to neglect the healthful foods nature offers, and we pay a price for that."[6] In most other cultures where dietary intake of healthy foods is a staple, menopause is a symptomless event. However, in the United States, with its reliance on processed, packaged fast foods, approximately 50% of women experience the mood swings and hot flashes of menopause.

How do you avoid the symptoms of menopause? Maintain a healthy diet supplemented with natural progesterone when indicated. However, it is very hard living in the Midwest to get the proper nutrition from even the healthiest foods. A major problem in the Midwest is that for three-fourths of the year, fruit and vegetables must be shipped in, therefore losing much of their nutrients in transit. I have seen many women go through menopause symptomless when they maintain proper levels of natural progesterone and eat a healthy diet.

Progesterone and Provera

There are two types of progesterone supplements available—natural progesterone and synthetic progesterone. Synthetic progesterone, such as Provera, resembles natural progesterone but has been chemically altered in order to be

Figure 7: A Comparison of a Natural Hormone (Natural Progesterone) and a Synthetic Hormone (Provera)

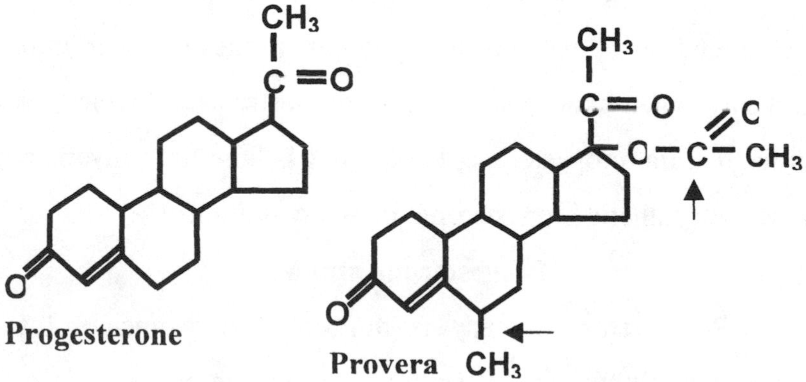

The difference between the natural hormone, progesterone, and the synthetic version, Provera, is illustrated in this diagram. The arrows in the Provera illustration point out the additional side chains added to progesterone. These added chains make Provera a foreign substance in the body, leading to an increased risk of adverse effects.

patented (see Figure 7). The body has receptors specifically for natural progesterone. There are no receptors in the body specifically for the synthetic forms of progesterone. This is why the natural form of a hormone like progesterone will always prevail—it has exact sites in the body waiting for it, while the synthetic forms do not. The synthetic forms act like a foreign substance to the body.

If the human body is accustomed to natural progesterone and has receptors of natural progesterone, doesn't it make sense to use natural progesterone versus a chemically altered form of progesterone? Researchers compared natural progesterone with synthetic progesterone and found better results with symptoms, lipid profiles, and side-effect profiles with natural progesterone.[7] I have found most patients on synthetic progestins will improve markedly when changed to natural progesterone. In fact, once I studied natural progesterone, I could not fathom how anyone could prescribe synthetic progesterone for any condition.

Progesterone and Men

Progesterone therapy is not only for women. Just as women benefit from small amounts of testosterone, men can also benefit from small amounts of progesterone. I have found natural progesterone effective for treating a variety of conditions in men including cardiovascular disorders, prostate problems (particularly prostatitis and benign prostatic hypertrophy), fatigue, autoimmune diseases, decreased libido, and others. In fact, most men that suffer from coronary artery disease will have a suppressed progesterone level and will improve when using small amounts of natural progesterone. I recommend using low doses of natural progesterone in men, from 2-10mg/day, while following serum levels.

DOSAGE

Natural progesterone is available in oral and transdermal preparations. I usually recommend a transdermal preparation because its absorption appears to be better than in the pill form. I recommend using U.S.P. grade micronized progesterone, typically derived from plants, and formulated by a compound pharmacist. I use strengths from 2-10% applied to the skin. I recommend you seek advice from a health care professional skilled in the use of natural hormones that can monitor your pre and post levels.

SIDE EFFECTS

There are few potential side effects of progesterone therapy. The most common side effects I have observed with natural progesterone are occasional breast tenderness and acne. These are usually dose-related problems and be easily remedied by adjusting the dose of natural progesterone.

NUTRITIONAL SUPPORT FOR THE OVARIES

A proper diet is the mainstay. Fresh fruits and vegetables are essential. Eliminate caffeine and drink adequate amounts of water. The ovaries require an adequate iodine intake to function optimally. Seafood is an excellent source of iodine, as is Celtic Sea Salt. The following supplements are helpful: Vitamin C-3,000mg/day, Vitamin D-400I.U./day, Calcium Citrate-1,000mg/day and Magnesium Chelate-400mg/day.

A WORD OF CAUTION

Health food stores may advertise products developed from yams as having natural progesterone-like effects on the body. It is impossible for the body to convert the chemicals in the yam to an active hormone such as progesterone. Unless natural progesterone is added to the product, the body will be unable to derive any progesterone benefits from it.

[1] Rossignol, A.M. Caffeine-containing beverages and premenstrual syndrome in young women,. American Journal of Public Heath. 1990;80:1106-10

[2] Prior, F.C. Progesterone as a bone trophic hormone. Endocrine Reviews. 18990;11:386-398

[3] Lee, John. IBID

[4] Lee, John. IBID

[5] Coenen, C.M., et al. Changes in androgens during treatment with four low-dose contraceptives. Contraception, March, 1996;53(3):171-6

[6] Lee, John. Natural Progesterone. The Multiple Roles of a Remarkable Hormone. BLL Publishing. 1993

[7] Hargrove, J.T., et al. Menopausal hormone replacement therapy with continuous daily oral micronized estradial and progesterone. OB&Gyn, 1989;71:606-612

Chapter 7

Natural Estrogens

Introduction

A difficult decision women have to make is whether to use estrogen for hormone replacement therapy. This is a very controversial topic. One must weigh the benefits of estrogen, which include providing relief from hot flashes as well as slowing down the rate of osteoporosis, versus the potential side effects such as an increased risk of endometrial cancer and, most likely, an increased risk of breast cancer. This chapter will explain the risks and benefits of estrogen replacement therapy and offer you a safer, more natural approach.

Estrogen is produced primarily in the ovaries. It is produced in a cyclical fashion in a menstruating woman. In a typical 28-day cycle, estrogen is produced in both the first half of the cycle known as the follicular phase, and in the second half of the cycle known as the luteal phase. Please refer to Figure 6, page 94 for more information. There are three different types of estrogens manufactured by the body: estrone, estradiol and estriol. Each of these different types of estrogen have very different properties in the body. Jonathan Wright M.D., a pioneer in natural therapies, measured the serum levels and urinary excretion of the three estrogens and reported that of the three types of estrogen measured, 80% was estriol, 10% was estrone and 10% was estradiol. If we're going to give estrogen replacement therapy to a woman, doesn't it make sense to give it in the same proportions as naturally made in the body? Unfortunately, traditional medicine's approach to estrogen replacement is not even close to these proportions.

Conventional estrogen replacement therapy usually consists of using synthetic derivatives of estrogen. Premarin, which is the most common synthetic estrogen product in use today, is a horse-derived estrogen complex, consisting primarily of estrone. Estrace, another common synthetic estrogen hormone, contains 100% estradiol. Neither contains the three forms of estrogen-- estriol, estrone and estradiol--in the percentages that are found naturally in the human body. Common sense would argue that to achieve the greatest benefit from estrogen replacement therapy, we should try to mimic the body's own production of estrogen. In other words, we should use the same proportions of estriol, estrone and estradiol normally produced in the body. A natural estrogen preparation has been formulated by Dr. Wright and is known as Triest. Triest is made from plant products and has the same chemical structure of the three types of estrogen produced in the human body. Triest mimics the body's own production of estrogens by containing 80% estriol, 10% estradiol and 10%

estrone. I believe that using Triest as compared to a synthetic estradiol or estrone compound is a much safer and more effective method to replace estrogens in a woman.

Case Study

Menopausal Symptoms

Cynthia, 51 years old, complained of debilitating hot flashes. "These hot flashes come 20-30 times per day, and I can't sleep at night. If that weren't enough, I've become a beast to my family with mood swings and depression. I feel like I should be committed," she stated. She reported drinking four cups of coffee every day. Upon using triest and natural progesterone, her hot flashes quickly ameliorated. Cynthia reported having an increased energy level and a significant improvement in her mood swings and depression. She also reported that stopping her caffeine intake improved her symptoms.

Discussion

Among the three estrogens, estradiol is the greatest stimulator of breast tissue and may play a role in promoting breast cancer. Estriol has the least stimulating effect on breast tissue and may be protective against breast cancer. In fact, the ratio of activity of estradiol and estriol in stimulating the breast tissue is 1000:1.[1] Two decades ago, research studies found estradiol and estrone increased one's risk of breast cancer, whereas estriol was protective.[2]   Estriol has also been shown to inhibit the breast cancer effect of estradiol in mice.[3]   An article in the Journal of the American Medical Association declared, "Estriol may not only be non-carcinogenic, but indeed anti-carcinogenic."[4]   Conventional estrogen replacement, which uses primarily estradiol or estrone, frequently causes endometrial (i.e., uterine) tissue to proliferate and produce a condition known as endometrial hyperplasia. This has not been observed with estriol therapy.[5]

Estrogen therapy is very successful in relieving the symptoms of menopause, including hot flashes, depression and mood swings.   Estrogen therapy does help slow down the progression of osteoporosis but does not reverse or prevent it. Unopposed estrogen therapy, (i.e. taking estrogen without taking progesterone), which is commonly prescribed by conventional doctors when a woman has had a hysterectomy, does have significant risks including: increasing the risk for blood clotting and fluid retention, promoting fat synthesis and the growth of uterine fibroids, as well as increasing the risk of endometrial cancer and possibly breast cancer.[6]

Conventional hormone replacement therapy always includes synthetic estrogen. Synthetic progesterone (i.e., Provera) is added to the regimen to help prevent uterine cancer. If a woman has had a hysterectomy she is not given Provera. This is a tragic mistake. No estrogen, whether natural or synthetic, should ever be taken without the balancing effect of natural progesterone.   I believe that the use of unopposed estrogens in conventional

108

hormone replacement therapy has been partially to blame for the epidemic rates of breast cancer found in this country.

When my patients who do not have a uterus question their gynecologists about the need for progesterone, oftentimes a gynecologist will comment that 'you don't need progesterone if you don't have a uterus'. That argument does not hold water. There are progesterone receptors throughout the body, including the bones, heart, liver, brain and other areas. Due to the overexposure of estrogens in the environment (from conventionally raised animals, pesticides, plastics, etc.), natural progesterone is necessary to help balance out the estrogen excess we are all exposed to.

Though I employ natural estrogens in my practice, I do so infrequently. This is because we live in a society of estrogen excess. There are exogenous estrogens, known as xenoestrogens, found in our environment that mimic estrogen's activity and can stimulate estrogen receptors in the body. Dr. Majid Ali, president of the American Academy of Preventive Medicine states, "We live in the age of estrogen overdrive...due to the chemicals that have estrogen-like effects."[7] These compounds are petrochemical derivatives commonly found in pesticides and plastics and may be responsible for the high rate of breast cancer and hysterectomies present today. These high hysterectomy rates are closely tied to the high rate of estrogen dependent fibroid tumors.[8] Fibroid tumors, as stated in the last chapter, develop from estrogen stimulation of the uterine tissue. Other known estrogen-dependent conditions include: endometriosis, endometrial cancer, and possibly breast cancer. In light of the above estrogen-dependent conditions, and as the environmental levels of xenoestrogens continue to grow, I do not use natural estrogens routinely in my practice. I primarily use them for women suffering from menopausal symptoms such as hot flashes, in which case they are extremely effective.

It is true that estrogen has been shown to retard osteoporosis. Contrary to what most physicians claim, estrogen therapy does not reverse or improve existing osteoporosis. In Harrison's Book of Internal Medicine, estrogens are noted "not capable of restoring bone mass."[9] I feel it is safer and more efficacious to use a combination of natural progesterone, DHEA and natural testosterone (covered in Chapter 8) along with nutritional supplements and dietary and lifestyle changes to treat osteoporosis. Dr. Lee examined the difference in bone mineral density in 63 females using progesterone supplementation, estrogen treatment, and a control group (i.e. without hormone treatment). His results showed that only natural progesterone can increase bone mass and therefore reverse osteoporosis.[10]

Dosage

Triest comes in pill or cream form. I generally use the cream, starting with 1.25mg and titrating the dosage until symptoms improve. I have observed that the cream form is easily absorbed through the skin.

Side Effects

Side effects of using estrogen compounds include increasing the risk of developing fibroid tumors, endometriosis, endometrial cancer, and possibly breast cancer. In addition, vaginal bleeding, high blood pressure, nausea, vomiting, headaches, fluid retention and glucose imbalances may occur with the use of estrogen compounds. Although I have not witnessed any major side effects with using natural estrogens, proper monitoring by a knowledgeable health care provider is necessary.

Nutritional Support for the Ovaries

Since estrogen, like progesterone is produced in the ovaries, the nutritional support is similar. A proper diet is the mainstay. Fresh fruits and vegetables are essential. Phytoestrogens, which are compounds found naturally in food, can stimulate the body's own estrogen receptors. Phytoestrogens are found in soy products and herbal products like Dong Quai and Black Cohosh. An adequate intake of phytoestrogens will minimize the symptoms of estrogen deficiency. In Asian countries, where the intake of fermented soy products* is very high, women suffer virtually no adverse symptoms of menopause. Phytoestrogens contain compounds that have no propensity to increase the risk of breast cancer, and many studies show that they may reduce the risk for cancer. Eliminate caffeine and drink adequate amounts of pure water per day. Eat iodine-containing foods including seafood and Celtic Sea Salt to satisfy the iodine requirements of the ovaries. Also the following supplements are helpful: Vitamin C 3000mg/day, Vitamin D 400 I.U./day, Calcium Citrate 1500mg/day and Magnesium Chelate 400mg/day.

*Most soy products in the United States are the non-fermented soy products. These products should be used sparingly, as they may inhibit thyroid function.

[1] Documenta Geigy, Scientific Tables sixth edition; pg 493.

[2] Lee, John. IBID, 40

[3] Lemon, H.M., et al. 1966 Reduced estriol excretion in patients with breast cancer prior to endocrine therapy. JAMA 196:1128-1136

[4] Follingstad, Alvin. Estriol, the forgotten Estrogen? JAMA 1/2/78 Vol. 239, No.1 pg. 29-30

[5] Gaby, Alan. *Preventing and reversing osteoporosis*. Prima Publishing. 1994

[6] Lee, John. IBID. 54

[7] Ali, Majit. *RDA, Rats, Drugs and Assumptions*. Life Span Press 1995

[8] Reported in an article, "In a culture of hysterectomies, many question their necessity." New York Times 2/17/97

[9] *Harrison's Book of Internal Medicine*, McGraw-Hill Book Company. 1989

[10] Lee, John Ibid 58

Chapter 8

Natural Testosterone

Introduction

Natural testosterone, when used prudently, is a very important part of hormone balancing in men and women. Testosterone is one of the major regulators of sugar, fat and protein metabolism in the body. Testosterone is the main hormone produced by the testicles in the man, with smaller amounts produced by the adrenal glands. In women, testosterone is produced in the ovaries and the adrenal glands. Women produce testosterone in much smaller amounts as compared to men. There are two forms of testosterone currently available: natural testosterone and synthetic testosterone. Natural testosterone is made from plant products and has the same chemical structure of testosterone that is produced in the human body. I have found natural testosterone very safe and effective in treating the above conditions.

Case Studies

Coronary Artery Disease

Perhaps the most stunning evidence for the use of natural testosterone is in treating coronary artery disease--the number one killer in the United States. Many millions of dollars are spent in this country treating heart disease with high-tech procedures like bypass surgery and balloon angioplasty, neither of which addresses the underlying problem(s). I believe one of the main components of coronary artery disease is a hormonal imbalance. This hormonal imbalance often includes low testosterone production as well as hypothyroidism. The link between coronary artery disease and hypothyroidism was addressed in Chapter 3. Furthermore, I have yet to see a severe coronary artery disease patient who did not have a significantly depressed testosterone level. Nor have I seen a cardiologist check levels of testosterone in such a patient.

My father, Ellis, is one such example. He had his first myocardial infarction (MI) or heart attack at age 42 and his first bypass surgery at age 50. Ellis' second bypass occurred at age 58. He had an angioplasty at age 60. Ellis never had his testosterone level checked during this entire time, yet he saw one of the best cardiologists in the area. He suffered from frequent bouts of angina throughout this time period, and I never recall him looking or acting well as I was growing up. Furthermore, his cholesterol levels were very high, usually in the 300's and virtually unresponsive to medications. When he was 63-years-old, I checked his testosterone level and found it to be extremely low at 1.5 ng/m (the normal range for men is 3-9 ng/ml). I placed him on Armour thyroid hormone for a low thyroid state, and natural testosterone due to his low levels. Since that time, he had virtually no symptoms of heart disease and, more importantly, he has never felt or looked better. Furthermore, his cholesterol level fell to less than 200mg/dl, and my father did NOT watch his diet, much to my consternation. After my parents took a trip with their high school friends Donna and Leonard, I received a phone call from Donna. She asked me what I was prescribing for my father. When I asked her why, she replied, "David, I haven't seen your father look this good in 30 years, I want to give Leonard the same thing." I believe my father may have been able to avoid much of his heart disease if he had been placed on natural hormones earlier in his life.

There are numerous studies linking atherosclerosis and coronary artery disease to low testosterone levels. A study by researchers from Columbia University's College of Physicians and Surgeons found those with low concentrations of testosterone in the blood were more likely to have atherosclerosis documented by angiography.[1] Moller, a Danish physician, found that 83% of patients' cholesterol levels fell significantly while taking testosterone. On average, the cholesterol level after testosterone was 74% of the pretreatment condition.[2] I'm sure these patients felt a lot better on this therapy compared to conventional medicine's approach of cholesterol-lowering medications and their side effects which include nausea, abdominal pain, gall bladder disease, a decreased libido, liver problems, and others. Several studies document low testosterone levels associated with high triglycerides and LDL cholesterol, which is thought to promote atherosclerosis. Other studies have shown that normal testosterone levels are associated with increased HDL cholesterol, which is thought to protect against atherosclerosis. In my practice, through the use of natural hormones like natural testosterone, I have witnessed the same type of results that my father experienced: a lowering of cholesterol levels and an improvement in the symptoms of coronary artery disease. These results are seen over and over in my practice. I believe that anyone who suffers from coronary artery disease should have a testosterone level checked just as quickly as a physician would investigate a cholesterol level. When low testosterone levels are adequately treated, many times coronary artery disease will improve.

Autoimmune Disorders: Lupus

Jackie, age 47, was diagnosed with lupus at age 35. She reported symptoms of joint and muscle pain, muscle wasting, difficulty concentrating and always feeling an overwhelming fatigue. "I just feel like I am slowly wasting away," she claimed. Her physician was treating her with Prednisone, a synthetic steroid hormone. Her testosterone level was so low, it was not even measurable in my lab. Upon taking 5mg of natural testosterone, she noticed an improvement in all of the above symptoms. Jackie claimed, "I feel so much better. I definitely have a higher energy level and I even look younger." Her testosterone level improved to a healthy .7 ng/ml, with normal levels for women ranging from .3-.8ng/ml. Jackie was also found to be hypothyroid and to have low levels of progesterone and DHEA. She noted improvement when treated with each of these natural hormones. One and one-half years later, she feels her disease has stopped progressing and may actually be reversing itself. Furthermore, she has been able to stay off all high dose steroid treatments, thus avoiding the negative side effects associated with steroids, such as osteoporosis, weight gain, etc.

In one study, females with active lupus were found to have significantly lower testosterone levels than those with inactive disease. The authors concluded that low levels of androgens, which include testosterone and DHEA, were thought to play a role in the development of autoimmune disease.[3] I have yet to see a patient ill from lupus or another autoimmune disease that does not have significantly depressed testosterone and DHEA levels. Furthermore, these patients often have lowered thyroid and ovarian function. Most people suffering from autoimmune disorders will respond favorably to physiologic replacement of natural hormones.

Fatigue and Low Libido

Natural testosterone replacement is a must for most women who have had a hysterectomy, either with or without removal of the ovaries. Testosterone is produced in the ovaries and the adrenal glands. After a hysterectomy, most women have an extremely low testosterone level.

Joan, at 48 years old, came to me complaining of extreme fatigue. She had a hysterectomy and removal of her ovaries due to fibroid tumors. Fibroid tumors, as explained in Chapter 6, are benign growths in the uterine wall and are thought to be due to a condition of estrogen excess. Joan claimed, "After my hysterectomy, I just haven't felt the same. My energy level has gone way down and I can barely get out of bed each morning. My doctor told me the only thing I would need is estrogen. I have tried three different (synthetic) estrogen pills and patches and could not tolerate any of these. They made me feel spacey and upset my stomach. In addition, my sex drive has gone to zero and my husband is totally frustrated. My doctor told me my libido would take time to return, but it is going nowhere." Joan had an extremely low testosterone level--less than 0.1ng/ml (normal .3-.8ng/ml). Furthermore, her progesterone level was almost zero (remember it used to be produced by her ovaries before they were removed), and her DHEA level was very low at 357ng/ml (normal for women 2000-3000ng/ml). Upon replacing these depleted

122

hormones, using natural testosterone, progesterone and DHEA, her symptoms immediately improved. After two months, Joan commented, "I am beginning to feel like my normal self again. My energy level is tremendously improved and my libido is improving. I only wish I had taken natural hormones earlier." Approximately six months after beginning the hormone replacement therapy, Joan reported that she felt as healthy as she did prior to her hysterectomy.

Diabetes

Testosterone is also of great benefit for patients with diabetes. I have found through using physiologic replacement doses of natural testosterone, diabetic patients are able to maintain much lower blood sugars and decrease insulin requirements.

Al, a 67-year-old insulin dependent diabetic suffered from poor blood sugar control and angina (i.e., chest pain). Upon taking natural testosterone, he found he needed much less insulin-- 20% less than he had been taking previously. Al was more excited about the other benefits of testosterone. He said, "I haven't felt any sexual desire in over 15 years. I thought that part of me was dead. It really is a wonderful surprise to have some sexual desire and ability return." Al has also found the energy to start exercising and his wife reports he is a happier, more contented person. Furthermore, his angina has almost totally disappeared.

Testosterone has also been shown to be effective for the complications of diabetes including diabetic retinopathy[4], gangrene, and peripheral vascular disease[5]. Moller describes outstanding results of testosterone therapy in treating claudication (i.e., leg pain when walking), gangrene, peripheral vascular disease, ulcerations and osteomyelitis (an infection which spreads to the bone and is often seen in diabetics), where patients were deemed to have diseases untreatable by surgery.[6] I wonder how many patients that have undergone bypass operations, either for heart disease or peripheral vascular disease, have ever had their testosterone level checked? Testosterone therapy can be a life and limb saving treatment option for these patients.

Chemotherapy

Testosterone therapy should be a high priority for any person who has received chemotherapy. Chemotherapeutic agents are poisons designed to kill highly active cancer cells. Unfortunately, highly active "regular" cells are also killed in this process. Some of the most highly active cells in the body reside in the hormone glands. I have found that although all of the hormones may be affected by chemotherapy, testosterone seems to be particularly affected, especially in men. In women, the ovarian hormones, estrogen and progesterone as well as testosterone are similarly affected.

Jimmy, age 19, was diagnosed with leukemia at age eight. He received chemotherapy treatments for two years and has been disease free since then. He presented with unrelenting fatigue and no libido. Needless to say, this is an upsetting condition for a 19 year old. Jimmy was found to be low thyroid via blood work and had basal temperatures that averaged 96.6 degrees. His fatigue

124

did improve somewhat on thyroid, but he received the most improvement from natural testosterone therapy. His initial testosterone level was 1.7ng/ml (normal for men 3.0-10ng/ml). Jimmy's testosterone level improved to a healthy 9.0ng/ml on 120mg of natural testosterone per day. "My sex drive was zero after the chemotherapy. Taking the natural testosterone made a huge improvement in my libido. Now I feel much more like a healthy 19 year old male instead of feeling like an old man," Jimmy commented.

Aging

Natural testosterone is also known to improve many signs of aging including a loss of muscle mass, an increase in fatigue, and a loss of libido.

George, a 64 year old maintenance supervisor, came to see me and complained of feeling fatigued all of the time. "I barely have enough energy to get through my job. Everything feels like a chore now." His wife accompanied him to the visit and claimed, "He has no energy to do anything. After work, he will fall asleep early in the evening. We have no sex life because he no longer has the energy or the interest." George appeared older than his age and I had to prod him to answer my questions. When I checked his testosterone level, it was very low at 1.5ng/ml (normal for men 3-10ng/ml). Upon taking 100mg of natural testosterone, George felt like he had become a new person. "I feel like I've been given 15 years back. My muscles no longer ache after work and I can get so much more accomplished during the day. The best part is that my sexual drive has returned. I thought that it was gone forever. I didn't realize how depressed I had felt until I started to feel better." Now, when George comes in for his office visits he is no longer sullen and always has a smile on his face. His wife was so impressed at George's progress that she became my patient and was also treated with natural testosterone. She also had an improvement in her energy level and felt much younger than her age.

Congestive Heart Failure

Bruce, 77 years old, was well until he had a heart attack two years ago. He had bypass surgery one year ago. Shortly after that, he developed congestive heart failure. Bruce's energy level had been steadily declining and he was suffering from worsening shortness of breath. "I have had constant chest pain since the surgery. Every day I am reminded of that surgery," he said. When I examined Bruce, he had very poor muscle tone. His testosterone level was very low at 270ng/dl. He was also found to have other hormone imbalances. Bruce was treated with a combination of natural testosterone, natural progesterone and DHEA along with vitamins, minerals and herbs. His testosterone level improved to a healthy 775ng/dl. About 6 weeks later, Bruce wrote me a letter that stated:

> "During the past two to three weeks, I have noticed a remarkable improvement in the way that I feel. The tightness and twinges of pain in the area of my heart have completely disappeared. I also have not had any shortness of breath, which was a problem prior

to this. Your program has far exceeded any expectations that I might have had."

The medical literature supporting the use of testosterone to treat congestive heart failure is vast. I believe every individual with congestive heart failure should be evaluated and treated for hormonal imbalances, particularly testosterone insufficiency.

Discussion

The discussion of testosterone brings thoughts of huge body builders taking anabolic (i.e., muscle and tissue building) steroids to artificially bulk up. When taken in extremely large doses, testosterone does promote the growth of huge muscles and aggressive, even violent behavior. In addition, large doses of testosterone can lead to the development of hypertension, baldness, acne and other deleterious side effects. However, in physiologic replacement doses--small doses that will not shut off the body's own production of the hormone--these negative side effects will not occur. In fact, I have found testosterone to be one of the most beneficial hormone replacement treatments for men as well as for women.

Testosterone therapy may reverse prostate growth and PSA levels. PSA is a blood test that, when elevated, may indicate an enlarged prostate gland or prostate cancer. Testosterone replacement therapy was found not only to lower PSA levels in men, but also to reverse the growth of the prostate gland. The researchers commented, "These findings suggest that testosterone {replacement} in middle-aged and older men with some clinical features of age-related {testosterone} deficiency can retard or reverse prostate growth…"[7]

As with the other hormones mentioned in this book, I recommend a natural form of testosterone. My reasoning is the same as previously presented in the other chapters. In order to get the maximum benefit from hormonal replacement therapy, it is important to try and mimic the body's own production of its hormones. I have found natural testosterone extremely safe and effective. In the United States, conventional testosterone therapy is frequently used with the patentable methyltestosterone, which has been found to be carcinogenic.[8]

Dosage

As I have indicated, I only use natural testosterone because it more closely mimics the body's own production of testosterone versus the synthetic derivatives of testosterone. Doses for women usually average 2-10mg per day. For men, doses usually range from 40-120mg per day. I prefer to use testosterone in cream form, as it is well absorbed through the skin. I recommend using USP grade micronized natural testosterone made by a compounding pharmacist.

Side Effects

Doses of testosterone that are too high can lead to the development of hypertension, acne, hair loss, anger, and mood swings. I have not observed any major negative effects using physiologic replacement doses of natural testosterone. There is concern that testosterone could adversely affect prostate cancer. I do not recommend any testosterone therapy for a patient who has a diagnosis of prostate cancer. This must be discussed with your physician. Taking an herb, saw palmetto, may block any possible negative effect of testosterone on the prostate by stopping the conversion of testosterone to dihydrotestosterone. Dihydrotestosterone is thought to cause the excess growth of the prostate gland.

Nutritional Support

In men taking testosterone, I recommend saw palmetto extract, for the reasons explained above. Vitamin C 3000mg/day and Vitamin E 400-800I.U. per day are also helpful for promoting testosterone production.

[1] Fackelmann, K.A. Science News, May 28, 1994;145:340

[2] Moller, Jens *Cholesterol, Interactions with Testosterone and Cortisol in Cardiovascular Diseases.* Springer-Verlag, 1987.

[3] Lahita, RG. Increased oxidation of testosterone in systemic Lupus erythematosus. Arthritis Rheum. 1983;26:1517-1521

[4] Douglass, William Campbell Second Opinion Newsletter. Vol. V. No. 3, March, 1995

[5] Moller, J, et al. *Testosterone Treatment of Cardiovascular Diseased, Principles and Clinical Experiences.* Springer-Verlag, 1984

[6] Moller, J. IBID

[7] Pechervsky, A.V., et al. Int. Androl. 2002. Apr;25(2):119-25

[8] Nutrition and Healing Newsletter, Vol. II No. 12, 1995

Chapter 9

Melatonin

Introduction

Anyone who has walked into a bookstore has seen numerous books touting the hormone 'melatonin' as a cure-all. Melatonin is a hormone secreted from the pineal gland, located in the brain. Melatonin is able to enter every cell of the body. It is made from an amino acid called tryptophan. Tryptophan is converted into serotonin, which is an important neurotransmitter thought to be associated with depression. Serotonin is converted into melatonin. High levels of tryptophan can be found in the following foods: fish, lamb, chicken, turkey and pumpkin seeds.

Case Study

Howard, 70 years old, complained of increased difficulty sleeping. He said, "I wake up four to five times per night. Sometimes I have to urinate, other times I just wake up. I used to sleep soundly all the time. It is very frustrating not to be able to get a good night's sleep." Howard tried over-the-counter sleeping agents to no avail. Upon taking 1mg of melatonin one hour before bedtime, he noticed an immediate improvement. He began getting up only once at night and reported his sleep quality was much better. "I haven't had dreams in ages, but now I remember all my dreams," Howard commented.

It is well known that melatonin can enhance the dream state. People routinely report more vivid dreams and usually find this a positive aspect of melatonin while about 10% of people taking melatonin report having nightmares. Melatonin supplementation will usually produce a deeper, more satisfying sleep. Upon taking melatonin, I have had more than one male patient tell me that he gets up fewer times at night to urinate. It is common for aging men to have to urinate throughout the night due to an enlarged prostate. Does melatonin keep men from getting up as much during the night because they have a deeper sleep or does melatonin have a direct effect on the prostate? Future studies need to be undertaken to answer this important question.

Discussion

The pineal gland regulates the circadian rhythm, otherwise known as our 24-hour biological clock, with the secretion of melatonin. At night, the pineal gland becomes activated and begins secreting melatonin, peaking between 2 a.m. and 4 a.m. Light, sensed through receptors in the eyes, inhibits the production of melatonin. Therefore, any light sensed by the eyes will shut off the production of melatonin.[1]

Melatonin levels, along with DHEA (Chapter 5) and human growth hormone (Chapter 11), progressively decline as we age. Perhaps the trigger for aging occurs as the level of melatonin (or DHEA or human growth hormone for that matter) progressively declines. Physiologic doses of these hormones may have anti-aging properties. Aging mice were given melatonin in their drinking water, and researchers found the mice lived an average of 20% longer.[2] A similar result was verified by researchers three years later.[3] Figure 8 illustrates the progressive decline in melatonin levels as we age.

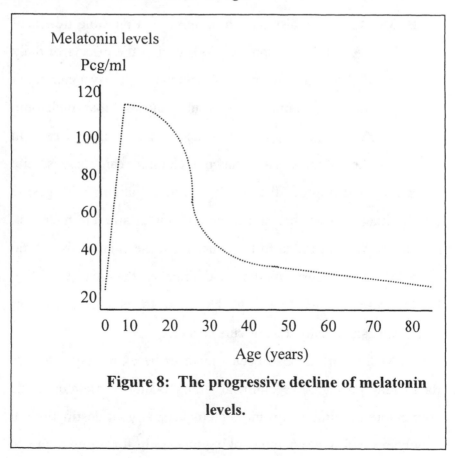

Figure 8: The progressive decline of melatonin levels.

One explanation for the aging process rests with free radicals. Free radicals are the byproducts of metabolism in our bodies. They are continually produced in our bodies, damaging cells and perhaps accelerating aging. Our bodies counter these free radicals with antioxidants, which act like vacuum cleaners, clearing our bodies of these free radicals. This breakdown and repair system is a continuous process in our bodies. Some examples of antioxidants include Vitamins C and E. Melatonin has been found to be a much more potent antioxidant than either Vitamin C or E.[4]

Melatonin has also shown promise as a possible treatment for cancer. A study was conducted observing the effects of daily injections of melatonin given to 54 patients with advanced colon cancer. After two months, the results showed that melatonin appeared to delay the progression of cancer in 44% of the cases. In addition, other studies have shown melatonin can increase life expectancy and improve the quality of life in patients with gastric cancer, lung cancer, breast cancer and metastatic brain cancer. Melatonin was not found to be a cure for these cancers, but it did seem to increase survival time and improve the quality of life. Further research will need to be done to elucidate whether melatonin can actually treat or cure cancer.

Melatonin has also been shown to be extremely effective for treating jet lag. I recommend taking 1-3mg of melatonin one hour before the time you want to go to sleep at your destination. It may be necessary to continue taking melatonin for a few nights in order to get the best results. If you are flying at night, I suggest taking melatonin 30 minutes before you wish to go to sleep.

I have also found melatonin to be effective for people who exercise late at night. Research has shown late night exercise (after 10p.m.) causes a suppressed melatonin release during sleep. On a personal note, taking 1mg of melatonin at bedtime has proven an immense benefit to me after playing tennis from 9 p.m. to 11p.m. No longer do I have difficulty falling asleep, nor do I feel as fatigued the next day. Another benefit I have noticed from taking melatonin is that my muscles are not as stiff the following day. This probably relates to the antioxidant effect of melatonin mentioned above.

Melatonin is also helpful for those undergoing detoxification programs. In order to ensure adequate antioxidant levels in the brain while undergoing detoxification, I recommend taking .5-1mg of melatonin at bedtime.

The elderly often have difficulty with interrupted sleep, which may be improved with physiologic replacement doses of melatonin. If you refer to Figure 8, you will see that the elderly have markedly diminished melatonin levels. For those that have difficulty sleeping, I always recommend a trial of melatonin.

Dosage

If one brand of melatonin does not work for you, I suggest you try another brand. It may be an absorption problem with one brand. I have seen numerous patients respond only to one particular brand of melatonin.

For anyone with difficulty sleeping, I suggest trying a small amount of melatonin. I recommend starting at low doses, generally around 1/2mg. Gradually increase the dose after two weeks if there is no response. I generally do not recommend using more than 3mg for sleep problems. The idea of replacing these hormones is to use physiologic doses, not large pharmacologic doses.

For jet lag, take melatonin about one hour before the actual time you want to go to sleep. You may have to take melatonin for several days to get the full benefit. I have found melatonin extremely helpful for traveling and usually only have to take it the first day of traveling to reset my internal time clock.

If you have next day fatigue, slowly decrease your dose until the fatigue disappears. This problem is easily remedied.

If you see no benefit from melatonin I generally recommend not taking it, as I do with all the natural hormones. Listen to your body--if it feels right, your body will let you know.

Side Effects

The only side effects I have observed with melatonin are next day grogginess and bad dreams. Decreasing the dose can often relieve the next day grogginess. As a personal note, when I take 3mg of melatonin, I am groggy for the entire next day. I do not observe this effect when I take .5mg of melatonin. If dreams become unpleasant when taking melatonin, I usually recommend either lowering the dose or discontinuing the melatonin.

I have found melatonin particularly safe. Many studies have been done with patients receiving large doses of melatonin and none of the studies have reported any significant side effects. However, because of the lack of research in using melatonin during pregnancy, I would not recommend women take it while pregnant or breast-feeding. Some practitioners do not recommend taking melatonin if the patient is suffering from an immune system disorder, such as lupus, rheumatoid arthritis, multiple sclerosis, Crohn's, ulcerative colitis, etc. These practitioners believe melatonin may adversely stimulate the immune system which may accelerate a disease state. However, I have not observed this negative reaction occurring. In fact, I have observed that a small amount of melatonin (see the previous section on dosage) has proven helpful in many of these disease states and I have not observed any major adverse effects.

Nutritional Support for Melatonin

Melatonin is manufactured from the amino acid tryptophan. Tryptophan is converted into serotonin, a neurotransmitter in the brain, and serotonin is converted into melatonin. Tryptophan is found in a variety of foods. As previously mentioned, diets high in chicken, beef, fish, lamb, turkey and pumpkin seeds contain high amounts of tryptophan and may promote the body's own production of melatonin. The B vitamins are important for the conversion of melatonin from tryptophan. I recommend one B Complex per day along with B6 50mg/day. L-tryptophan supplementation may also be helpful in promoting melatonin production.

Final Thoughts

I have found melatonin effective for about 60% of patients that have sleep difficulties. I think melatonin should be used along with the other natural hormones mentioned in this book when indicated. I have often observed that melatonin alone did not improve sleep, but with the addition of DHEA, melatonin became much more effective. Sometimes finding the right combination is a process of trial and error. Be patient and find the right treatment for you. The benefit of melatonin is surely worth the effort of finding what works for your body.

[1] Sahelian, Ray. <u>Melatonin, Natures Sleeping Pill</u>. Avery, 1995

[2] Maestroni, G, et al. Pineal melatonin, its fundamental immunoregulatory role in aging and cancer. Annals NY Acad. Sciences 521:140-8, 1988

[3] Pierpaoli,W, et al. the pineal control of aging: the effects of melatonin and pineal grafting on the survival of older mice. Annals NY Acad Sciences 621:291-313, 1991

[4] Hardeland R, et al. The significance of the metabolism of the neurohormone melatonin: antioxidative protection and formation of bioactive substances. Neuroscience and Biobehavioral Reviews 17: 347-57, 1993

Chapter 10

Hydrocortisone

Introduction

Hydrocortisone is a hormone produced in the adrenal glands--the same glands that produce DHEA. Adequate production of hydrocortisone is the body's major line of defense against stressful situations, including infections and injuries. When the body is placed under a stressful situation, one of the body's primary responses is to increase the output of hydrocortisone. Without this increased production of hydrocortisone the body is unable to adapt to the stressful situation. When there is not adequate production of hydrocortisone, there is an increased susceptibility to illness, such as the common cold, as well as longer recovery times and more severe infections from illness. In fact, adequate levels of hydrocortisone are necessary for the immune system to function properly and for the body to heal itself from illness or infection. For people who have deficient hydrocortisone production, physiologic replacement doses can improve the immune system and reverse many chronic conditions, without any serious side effects.

Case Study

Chronic Fatigue

Marsha, 35 years old, complained of chronic fatigue for five years. She was well until she got the flu and never recovered. Before she was ill, she was very active as an artist and enjoyed exercising daily. Marsha claimed, "Now when I exercise, I feel worse. After I do 20 minutes on the bike, I feel terrible. It takes me two days to recover." She also complained of feeling cold all the time and having very painful PMS and heavy bleeding with her periods. Marsha consulted with a doctor three years ago who tried her on thyroid hormone, but this actually made her symptoms worse. When I saw her in my office, Marsha looked older than her age. Her blood pressure was 90/56 lying down and fell to 80/50 standing up. A normal response should be for the blood pressure to increase upon standing. Whenever I see someone with an extremely low blood pressure, I always investigate the adrenal glands. A low blood pressure often reflects the adrenal glands producing subnormal levels of hydrocortisone. I frequently find that someone with a systolic blood pressure less than 100 is often fatigued and not feeling well. Proper adrenal gland functioning, including hydrocortisone production, is essential to maintaining a normal blood pressure. If the blood pressure is too low, tissues are not supplied with enough nutrients, causing muscle aches. In addition there is usually an inability to exercise, primarily because the body cannot pump enough blood to supply the muscles proper nutrients, as in Marsha's case. Marsha collected urine for 24 hours to assess her adrenal function. Her 24-hour urine test showed a dramatically low output of hydrocortisone. I have found that if thyroid therapy is given before the adrenal problem is addressed, many people like Marsha actually feel worse. Adequate hydrocortisone levels are necessary to promote the conversion of thyroid hormone from an inactive state (T4) to an active state (T3). Without the proper conversion taking place, thyroid supplementation can actually worsen someone's symptoms if the adrenal problems are not addressed. Upon placing Marsha on 15mg of hydrocortisone and 60mg of Armour thyroid, her symptoms rapidly cleared. Her blood pressure improved to 120/78 and she found she was able to exercise daily. Marsha said, "I can't believe the difference the hydrocortisone made in me. My energy level returned to normal and I feel like my old self again. In addition, now I can exercise and feel good afterwards." Again, this case illustrates the synergistic effects of using the natural hormones in combination with each other.

Discussion

Most physicians and lay people do not understand the benefits and importance of normal hydrocortisone production in the body. I was taught in medical school that the use of hydrocortisone-like products (e.g. Prednisone, a synthetic steroid product), were only to be used as a "last resort" to treat illness. The adverse side effects of using hydrocortisone medications were well known to me: promoting osteoporosis, obesity, hypertension, etc. What was not explained was that these negative side effects of hydrocortisone treatments only occur when these medications are used in excess of physiologic (i.e. small) replacement doses.

Dr. William Jeffries, Professor Emeritus at Case Western Reserve University, was a pioneer in developing the proper uses of physiologic replacement doses of hydrocortisone. Dr. Jeffries had over one hundred patient years of experience with using small physiologic replacement doses of hydrocortisone without any of the major side effects associated with the pharmacologic (i.e. large) doses. Again, it is necessary to explain the difference between physiologic and pharmacologic doses of hormones. A physiologic dose refers to a dosage necessary to maintain normal levels of a hormone. Physiologic doses are small enough so as not to shut off the body's own production of its hormones. On the other hand, large pharmacologic doses cause the body to sense there is too much of the hormone in circulation, resulting in the body decreasing its own production of the hormone. At this stage, the body becomes dependent on these large doses and negative side effects will begin to occur.

Some background information on normal hydrocortisone production is essential to understanding why the use of replacement doses of hydrocortisone is so effective. The adrenal glands are very sensitive to exogenous (i.e., outside the body) hydrocortisone intake. Under normal unstressed conditions, the adrenal glands produce the equivalent of approximately 40mg/day of hydrocortisone taken orally.[1] When one takes greater than 40 mg/day of hydrocortisone, the adrenal glands will cease production of this hormone, sensing too much hydrocortisone in the body. From this point on, one becomes dependent on these exogenous sources of hydrocortisone for survival, and negative side effects will occur. Dr. Jeffries found that physiologic replacement doses of 10-20mg of hydrocortisone per day do not cause the adrenal glands to cease production of their hormones and do not lead to the negative side effects mentioned with using the larger doses. In fact, physiologic doses bring a patient's low levels of hydrocortisone into a normal range and will help the body fight against infection or illness.

There is no better validation of a therapy than having it confirmed in an animal model. Dr. Alfred Plechner, a veterinarian has been treating hydrocortisone deficiency in dogs and cats for over 30 years. Dr. Plechner found that dogs and cats that had severe allergies and chronic illness often had adrenal problems whereby the adrenal glands did not produce enough hydrocortisone. This hypoadrenal state would lead to thyroid abnormalities and immune system malfunction. Ultimately, the endocrine abnormalities predispose the animals to autoimmune disorders, infections, and cancer.[2] This is the same pattern that I have observed in my human patients.

Trey, at 13 years old, was feeling her age. She developed arthritis in her hips and was losing her hair in large clumps. She was also suffering from anxiety and would have daily panic attacks. Through blood testing, Trey was diagnosed with an immune system imbalance (secondary to low Cortisol output by the adrenal glands) and hypothyroidism. When Trey was placed on natural hydrocortisone and thyroid hormone, all of her symptoms improved, almost immediately.

Trey is my dog. Trey was experiencing many of the same problems that I see in my own patients. When Trey's hormonal system was finally balanced with small amounts of natural hormones (hydrocortisone, DHEA, natural progesterone, pregnenolone and thyroid hormone) all of her symptoms vanished. Trey began acting as a youthful dog again, getting into the garbage, taking food from the children, etc. Trey is a perfect example of the positive benefits of using natural hormones to restore balance to the hormonal and immune systems.

There are many synthetic derivatives of hydrocortisone available for use today. Prednisone is the most commonly used synthetic hormone. However, as with the other hormones mentioned in this book, I believe we should strive to mimic the body's own production of hormones. Natural hydrocortisone is the name of the hormone that most closely mimics the adrenal glands' production of hydrocortisone. In treating a low adrenal state, I have achieved much better results with using natural hydrocortisone rather than other synthetic derivatives such as Prednisone. Natural hydrocortisone is available from a compounding pharmacist.

It is important to realize different hormones have different potencies. For example, 5mg of Prednisone, a synthetic derivative of hydrocortisone, is equivalent to approximately 20mg of hydrocortisone. When pharmacologic doses of Prednisone are used, (which are doses in excess of 10mg/day), the adrenal glands will, by a negative feedback mechanism, shut off their production of hormones due to the excess dose being taken. This is where the negative side effects such as hypertension, weight gain, osteoporosis, etc., will begin to appear. As long as physiologic doses of hydrocortisone are used, generally not exceeding 40mg/day, adrenal suppression will not occur and unwanted side effects will be avoided.

Dr. Barnes (from Chapter 3) felt that up to 40% of hypothyroid patients are found to be hypoadrenal as well. In my practice I have found a similar percentage of hypothyroid patients also suffer from hypoadrenalism. I have also observed that many hypothyroid patients will not improve until their low adrenal state is addressed, often with using physiologic replacement doses of hydrocortisone.

Dosage

For physiologic replacement doses of hydrocortisone, I do not recommend using doses greater than 40mg per day. This dose will not promote adverse effects and ensures the adrenal glands will not shut off their own production of hydrocortisone. The dose I generally use is 5mg of natural hydrocortisone three times per day with meals. I always check 24-hour urine levels for hydrocortisone output (via a total 17-hydroxy steroid level for 24 hours) before and after hydrocortisone therapy to monitor the output. Hydrocortisone dosages need to be closely monitored by a health care practitioner knowledgeable in the use of natural hormones.

Side Effects

The side effects of hydrocortisone and other steroids include the promotion of: weight gain, osteoporosis, atherosclerosis, blood sugar abnormalities and others. I have not observed any major side effects with using hydrocortisone in physiologic replacement doses--doses less than 40mg per day. The main side effect I have observed with a physiologic dose is a small weight gain, usually less than five pounds. Usually this weight gain will subside after one to two months of taking hydrocortisone.

Nutritional Support for the Adrenal Glands

I have found nutritional support to be very effective for low cortisol states. Herbal therapies, such as licorice root extract 600mg/day and Gotu Kola 50-100mg have been very helpful. These herbs are useful for building up the adrenal gland and stimulating hydrocortisone receptors in the body.[3] Vitamin supplementation includes Vitamin C- 3000mg/day (since the adrenal glands have the highest concentration of Vitamin C in the body), and Vitamin E- 400 I.U./day. Adrenal glandulars have also been helpful and are available at health food stores.

[1] Jeffries, William. Safe Uses of Cortisol. Charles C. Thomas, 1996

[2] Plechner, Alfred. An effective veterinary model may offer therapeutic promise for human conditions: roles of cortisol and thyroid hormones. Medical Hypotheses, in press.

[3] Mawrey, Daniel. The Scientific Validation of Herbal Medicine. Keats, 1986

Chapter 11

Human Growth Hormone

BENEFITS OF HUMAN GROWTH HORMONE

The beneficial effects of using physiologic doses of human growth hormone include improving and perhaps reversing many of the following signs of aging: thinning hair, wrinkled skin, loss of muscle tone, low resistance to stress, depression, low resistance to infection, poor healing of wounds, and varicose veins. Human growth hormone has also been shown to improve the following conditions: cardiac disease, fatigue, osteoporosis, and perhaps cancer.

Introduction

Human growth hormone is secreted by the pituitary gland, which is located in the center of the brain. It is named human growth hormone because its production peaks during the intense growth spurt of adolescence. Children lacking the proper production of human growth hormone will have an extremely short stature. Adults lacking human growth hormone have many signs of accelerated aging including: increased skin wrinkling, decreased energy levels, poor sexual function, increased body fat, and signs of osteoporosis. Furthermore, accelerated cardiovascular diseases are common in adults with human growth hormone insufficiency.

After the pituitary gland secretes human growth hormone, it causes the liver to secrete another hormone called insulin-like growth factor 1 or IGF-1 (illustrated in Figure 9). It is IGF-1 that is responsible for the effects human growth hormone has on the body. IGF-1 is easily measured in the blood, and is the most common measurement used to assess growth hormone status.   All levels of growth hormone mentioned in this book are measured as IGF-1 levels.

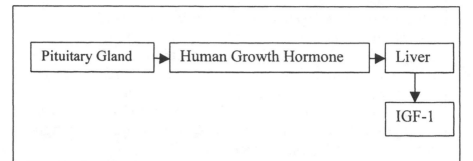

Figure 9: The release of human growth hormone from the pituitary, which leads to the release of IGF-1 from the liver.

CASE STUDIES

Aging and Fatigue

Veronica, age 44, was upset about some of the signs of aging she was experiencing. She said, "I seem to exercise more, yet I have a harder time holding my weight down. I cannot exercise with the same intensity I used to when I was younger. Also, I always feel fatigued, no matter how much sleep I get." In addition, Veronica suffered from painful, irregular periods. Due to her fatigue, she was having a hard time managing her business and taking care of her family. Her initial level of growth hormone was low at 132ng/ml. After taking human growth hormone for two months, her growth hormone level improved to a healthy 286ng/ml. Veronica was amazed at the improvement in her health.

"The change I feel already is amazing. My energy level has risen dramatically and now I feel like I used to feel when I was in my twenties. Fatty areas of my body are decreasing and my workouts are better than ever. My business is flourishing because I have so much energy to put into it," she claimed. In addition, Veronica's periods became regular and much less painful. She stated, "My family and friends think I look younger already and they are reading up on growth hormone."

Fibromyalgia

Frank, 34 years old, was suffering from fibromyalgia and reported feeling like an old man. Frank had been treated for hypertension for five years with Procardia, an antihypertensive medication. His blood pressure averaged 140/90, which is on the high side. In addition to feeling fatigued all of the time, Frank said, "I have pains all over my body, every day of my life. In fact, I cannot recall a day in my life since I was a teenager that I did not have back pains. Also, I have a constant pressure in the front of my chest. I have taken a lot of tests and seen many doctors and they all tell me that nothing is wrong. If that isn't enough, I always have pains running up and down my neck. Doctors keep telling me my muscles are "stressed out" but they have not given me anything to help." Frank used to be a pitcher in high school. After pitching a game, he was so sore that his mother and sister would ice down his back and chest for hours. Now, his wife and children constantly massage his back to try to keep it loose. "Also, I have *lost a tremendous amount of muscle strength over the years. My arms feel extremely weak and I can barely lift anything," he commented. When I examined Frank, I was surprised at his lack of muscle strength. Frank was a large man, six feet four inches tall, but he was very weak when I tested the strength of his muscles. Frank's initial growth hormone level was low at 121ng/ml. After taking human growth hormone for two months he reported, "I feel remarkably better. My energy level is starting to return to normal and my aches and pains are at least 80% better." After four months of growth hormone therapy, Frank went out of town for three days and forgot to take the growth hormone with him. He stated, "Now I know how much better I felt when I was taking growth hormone. On the second day after not taking my growth hormone, all of my aches and pains started to come back. In fact, I was doing so well on the growth hormone therapy that I had forgotten about my chest and back pain. When my pains started to come back, I knew I had to go back on the growth hormone right away. Now that I am taking growth hormone, my muscle strength is continuing to get better and I am able to work out daily because I have so much energy." Also, Frank's blood pressure has decreased to a healthy 130/70 and he has lowered his Procardia dose by half. Research has shown physiologic doses of human growth hormone restored muscle strength in 88% of patients taking it. In addition energy levels increased in 84% of those treated.*[1]

Muscle Weakness

Elaine, 64 years old, felt the signs of aging. "I want to feel like I did when I was younger. I work out two days per week and I stay very active, but I can't seem to build any muscle," she said. Elaine also complained about other signs of aging such as wrinkling of her skin, excess fat deposition and difficulty concentrating. "I used to be so sharp mentally. Now, it takes me forever to think of things. I am too young to grow old," she lamented. Elaine had researched growth hormone therapy on her own and wanted to try it. Her initial growth hormone level was low at 105ng/ml. When she was placed on human growth hormone therapy she noticed immediate improvements. "I feel like I am 20 years younger. My friends can no longer keep up with me. My skin is better and most of all my concentration is better. In fact, all of the signs of aging seem to have improved," she happily reported. Elaine now has enough energy to exercise four days per week. Elaine's growth hormone level rose to a healthy 250ng/ml.

Discussion

In adults, human growth hormone production gradually declines as one ages, as illustrated in Figure 10. This gradual decline parallels the age-related decline of DHEA (Chapter 5), natural testosterone (Chapter 8), melatonin (Chapter 9) and pregnenolone (Chapter 12). After age 20, human growth hormone levels fall by 50% approximately every seven years in a healthy, young population. Perhaps by raising levels of human growth hormone (as well as DHEA, melatonin, testosterone and the other hormones) to levels present at younger years, we can slow down or even reverse many of the signs and symptoms of aging. Supplementation of human growth hormone, along with the other natural hormones in this book, does appear to clinically reverse many of the signs of aging in most people who take it.

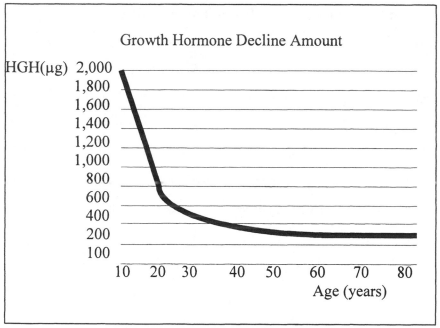

Figure 10: Human growth hormone decline as related to aging[2]

A study by Dr. Daniel Rudman, published in the New England Journal of Medicine showed that men who received six months of human growth hormone injections had improvements in almost every body area measured.[3] The improvements included:

1. An 8.8% increase in lean muscle mass.
2. A 14.4% decrease in body fat.
3. A 1.7% increase in bone density of the lumbar vertebrae.
4. A 7.1% increase in skin thickness.

Dr. Rudman concluded that the benefits of six months of human growth hormone replacement were equivalent to a reversal of 10-20 years of aging.[4] Dr. Rudman's work has been validated in many other studies and I have seen similar positive responses in my patients who use growth hormone.

Because growth hormone is an anabolic or tissue-building hormone (similar to testosterone), conditions that result in loss of tissue could theoretically be improved by human growth hormone supplementation. The use of physiologic doses of human growth hormone seems to improve many of these conditions including:

1. Osteoporosis. Studies have shown that adults deficient in growth hormone have lower bone mineral density.[5] Further studies have determined that growth hormone supplementation can increase bone mineral density.
2. Cardiovascular diseases. It has been shown that

human growth hormone supplementation has improved cardiomyopathy and congestive heart failure.[6] Human growth hormone supplementation should be the treatment of choice for these serious conditions.

3. <u>Signs of aging.</u> Growth hormone has been shown to reverse skin wrinkling, muscle loss, bone loss, thinning skin and other signs of aging.

Fibromyalgia is another chronic condition for which human growth hormone has been shown to be effective. Researchers have found that deficient growth hormone secretion is common among fibromyalgia patients. Of 50 fibromyalgia patients tested, 41 (84%) were found to be deficient in growth hormone secretion.[7] In my practice, I have found similar percentages of fibromyalgia patients with decreased growth hormone levels. Most of these patients will report significant improvement in their condition when growth hormone levels are raised.

Obesity has a negative correlation with growth hormone secretion. Typically the more obese an individual is, the less growth hormone will be secreted. Growth hormone therapy not only promotes fat loss but will also result in an increase in lean tissue (i.e. muscle).[8]

Physiologic doses of human growth hormone may hold promise for cancer treatments. In my experience, most patients with cancer have suppressed growth hormone levels. In fact, I have yet to see a patient ill from cancer that does not have a decreased growth hormone level. Decreased growth hormone levels have been reported in liver cancer,[9] endometrial (uterine) cancer,[10] and colon cancer.[11] One study on cancer patients showed that growth hormone supplementation reversed body wasting and promoted the growth of lean tissue.[12]

Large doses of human growth hormone, however may be cancer promoting. In acromegaly, a condition where the pituitary gland secretes excess amounts of growth hormone, there is an increased rate of cancer. On the other hand, the rate of human growth hormone production in acromegaly far exceeds the physiologic doses of growth hormone recommended in this book. Presently, there are no studies that indicate that physiologic (i.e., small) doses of human growth hormone promote cancer growth. Further research should be conducted to determine the potential benefits and hazards of using physiologic doses of growth hormone.

Supplementation of human growth hormone is somewhat limited by its cost. Human growth hormone is presently made by only a few pharmaceutical companies. It is manufactured using recombinant DNA technology, similar to the way insulin is manufactured. Often insurance companies will only reimburse for human growth hormone when it is used for children with human growth hormone deficiencies. Presently, the cost of using human growth hormone can run up to $5,000 per year. Due to the high cost, I have not prescribed human growth hormone as much as the other hormones mentioned in this book. However, I think human growth hormone is an important piece of the puzzle when treating the signs of aging or when treating many chronic diseases including cardiovascular disorders and fibromyalgia.

So how do you raise human growth hormone levels without incurring the large expense of using growth hormone? Exercise has been shown in numerous studies to enhance the body's natural release of human growth hormone. As a natural response to exercise, the body will secrete increasing amounts of human growth hormone. This is one of the primary reasons it is so important to exercise on a regular basis.

Natural hormones have also been shown to be effective at stimulating growth hormone release. Researchers found that DHEA supplementation could restore growth hormone production. The authors of the study point out that the increase in growth hormone levels was accompanied by "a remarkable increase in perceived physical and psychological well-being for both men and women.[13]All of the hormones covered in this book have been shown to increase growth hormone levels. I have found that using combinations of natural hormones is extremely effective at promoting elevated levels of human growth hormone in the body. This is yet another reason why these hormones should be used in combination to achieve the best results.

Nutritional supplementation can also promote elevated growth hormone levels. Amino acids such as arginine, lysine, ornithine, glutamine, glycine, tryptophan and tyrosine have been shown to improve growth hormone levels. Niacin has also been effective. These nutritional items also work better to raise growth hormone levels when used in combination rather than individually.

An interesting nutritional product, Gammanol Forte (manufactured by Biotics Research) can raise growth hormone levels by more than 50% in some people. Gammanol Forte contains gamma oryzanol, which is found in rice bran. I have completed an outcome study that showed that 8 of 11 women given Gammanol Forte (6 tabs per day) had growth hormone levels rise by an average of 45%. Although growth hormone levels do rise with some nutritional supplements (like Gammanol Forte), the best clinical response to elevated growth hormone levels occurs through the use of actual human growth hormone.

Dosage

Human growth hormone is given in injection form. It is given in doses of 0.05-1.5 I.U. per day in a subcutaneous injection, which is similar to an insulin injection. Growth hormone is best given in two divided shots per day, usually in the morning and at bedtime, which mimics the body's own rhythm of secreting growth hormone. Growth hormone, like all the other hormones mentioned in this book should be used in physiologic (i.e. small) doses only. Growth hormone can be measured in the blood as an IGF-1 test. I have found effective serum levels for IGF-1 range from 250-350ng/ml. All levels referred to in this book are IGF-1 levels.

Side Effects

One side effect of using human growth hormone is increasing the risk for acromegaly. Acromegaly is a condition where huge amounts of human growth hormone are secreted in the body resulting in a higher incidence of cardiac problems and premature death. Acromegaly is seen in athletes who take massive doses of human growth hormone and in other people who are born with a pituitary gland that erroneously secretes excess amounts of human growth hormone. Other adverse effects of human growth hormone include: carpal tunnel syndrome, achiness in the joints and muscles, and edema. These side effects were reported with high doses of human growth hormone and are almost nonexistent when using lower doses. Most of these side effects are easily reversible by lowering the dose. I have observed few adverse effects with using physiologic doses of human growth hormone.

Nutritional Support

Numerous studies have demonstrated a correlation between excess body fat and decreased hormone levels. The easiest way to naturally increase your production of human growth hormone is to exercise. A daily exercise regimen will stimulate the body to produce increased amounts of human growth hormone. I recommend moderate aerobic exercise of 30 minutes three to five times per week. An appropriate exercise regimen can be discussed with your health care provider. Amino acid supplementation has also been shown in numerous studies to raise human growth hormone levels. In addition, glutamine, in doses of two grams per day, has been shown to raise growth hormone levels.[14] Further, there is evidence that L-arginine and L-lysine raise growth hormone levels. These amino acids are best used in combination due to their synergistic effect in raising growth hormone levels. Niacin, in doses less than one gram per day, has also been shown to elevate growth hormone levels.

Final Thoughts

There is some concern that supplementation with human growth hormone may be stimulating to some cancer cells. There are some studies which show human growth hormone may be stimulating to leukemia and lymphoma cells in cultures. Other studies showed huge doses of human growth hormone in rats promoted tumor growth. However, there are many studies which show human growth hormone does not increase the risk of cancer and actually improves the functioning of the immune system. Because there is a concern of possible increased growth of cancer with human growth hormone supplementation, anyone with cancer must discuss human growth hormone therapy with his or her oncologist.

Human growth hormone, when used appropriately, is a very safe and effective way to improve health and reverse many of the signs of aging. As with all of the hormones mentioned in this book, it is important to seek care from a health care practitioner knowledgeable in the use of natural hormones.

[11] Klatz, Ronald. <u>Grow Young With HGH.</u> Harper Collins, 1995, p. 36

[2] Journal of NIH Research, Adapted from, April, 1995

[3] Rudman, Daniel, et al. Effects of growth hormone in men over 60years. New England Journal of Medicine, 323, 1-6, 1990

[4] Rudman, Daniel. IBID.

[5] Beshyah, S.A., et al. Abnormal body composition and reduced bone mass in growth hormone deficient hypopituitary adults. Clinical Endocrinology (42): 179-189, 1995

[6] Fazio, S., et al. A preliminary study of growth hormone in the treatment of dilated cardiomyopathy. New England Journal of Medicine. 334: 809-14, 1996.

[7] Article in Family Practice News. Fibromyalgia may have a growth hormone problem. Family Practice News. Vol. 27, No. 16. 8/25/97

[8] Rudman, Daniel, et al. IBID.

[9] Wing, J.R., et al. Hypoglycemia in hepatocellular carcinoma: Failure of short-term growth hormone administration to reduce enhanced glucose requirements. Metabolism, 40(5): 508-512.

[10] Rutanen, E.M., et al. Relationship between carbohydrate metabolism and serum insulin-like growth factor system in postmenopausal women: Comparison of endometrial cancer patients with healthy controls. Journal of Clinical Endocrinological Metabolism, 77 (1): 199-204.

[11] El Atiz., et al. Alterations in serum levels of insulin-like growth factors and insulin-like growth-factor-binding proteins in patients with colorectal cancer. Int. Journal of Cancer, 57 (4): 491-497, 1994.

[12] Wolf, R.F., et al. Growth hormone and insulin reverse net whole body and skeletal muscle protein catabolism in cancer patients. Annals of Surgery. 216(3): 80-290, 1992/

[13] Morales, A.J., et al. Effects of replacement dose of dehydroepiandrosterone in men and women of advancing age. J. Clin.Edocrinol. Metab. 1994;78(6):1360-7

[14] Welbourne, T. Increased plasma bicarbonate and growth hormone after oral glutamine load. American Journal of Clinical Nutrition. 61(1995): 1057-62

Chapter 12

Pregnenolone

> **BENEFITS OF PREGNENOLONE**
>
> The benefits of physiologic doses of pregnenolone include the treatment of the following conditions: arthritis, depression, fatigue states, memory loss and moodiness.

Introduction

Pregnenolone is a steroid hormone produced in the adrenal glands. Pregnenolone is often referred to as the "mother hormone", since it is the precursor hormone to all of the adrenal hormones (refer to Figure 4, page 61). It is formed from cholesterol and is necessary to produce other adrenal hormones including progesterone, DHEA, hydrocortisone, testosterone, and the estrogens. Pregnenolone is also produced in the brain. In fact, pregnenolone levels in the brain are much higher than they are in the peripheral tissues.[1] Pregnenolone has been shown to affect many of the neurotransmitters in the brain. Pregnenolone levels, like the other hormones mentioned in this book, decline with age. At age 75, there is a 65% reduction in pregnenolone production in the body as compared to levels at age 35.[2] I have found pregnenolone particularly useful in treating memory problems, fatigue and depression.

Case Studies

Chronic Fatigue Syndrome

Yolanda, age 47, suffered from chronic fatigue syndrome for many years. She became ill with the flu and never fully recovered. Yolanda was found to be hypothyroid and hypoadrenal. I treated her with physiologic doses of Armour thyroid, DHEA, natural progesterone and natural testosterone. Yolanda was thrilled with her progress, "I felt like I was dying before using the natural hormones. Now, I feel like my life is coming back." Though Yolanda's condition was much improved, she still found her memory was poor. "It feels like I have a cloud in my head. Before I became ill, my mind was "lightening-quick". Now, it seems as if it takes forever for my brain to finish a thought," she said. Though her thought processes were better on the natural hormones, they were not back to normal. When I checked a pregnenolone level on her, it did not measure (it was reported as <11Ng/ml). Upon taking 5mg of pregnenolone twice per day, her memory immediately improved. "After one week of the pregnenolone, the cloud lifted and I felt my mind return to normal. Now I feel as if I have regained all that I had lost," she claimed.

Discussion

Pregnenolone production, like DHEA, testosterone and the other hormones covered in this book, gradually declines as we age.

Physiologic replacement doses of pregnenolone are important for treating memory and mood problems, as well as depression. Animal studies have shown a benefit in memory in animals treated with pregnenolone (as well as other natural hormones such as DHEA and testosterone).[3] Studies have also indicated pregnenolone may be beneficial for treating arthritis.

I have observed extremely low levels of pregnenolone in people who suffer from chronic ailments, such as autoimmune disorders, chronic fatigue and depression. Often, small doses of pregnenolone have been beneficial for these conditions.

Pregnenolone (and DHEA) can help regulate the functioning of the immune system. Research has shown that physiologic doses of pregnenolone (and DHEA) can result in increased function of the immune system in rats.[4]

Pregnenolone is extremely safe. Though the studies on pregnenolone are few, rodent and human studies have failed to show any major side effects from taking large doses of pregnenolone. In one study, 525mg of pregnenolone taken daily for three months did not induce any apparent toxicity.[5] As with the other hormones covered in this book, I do not recommend taking large doses of pregnenolone. A small, physiologic replacement dose, used with appropriate supervision, is the safest, most effective way to use natural hormones.

Although I have found small doses of pregnenolone effective for improving the conditions listed above, it is not effective for everyone. Many people report no improvement with pregnenolone. I have found the best results with pregnenolone are achieved when it is used in combination with other natural hormones. Pregnenolone levels, like the other hormones covered in this book, need to be appropriately monitored.

Dosage

Though pregnenolone is available over the counter at health food stores, I recommend using pregnenolone that is made by a compounding pharmacist. I have found the doses of pregnenolone commonly available at health food stores too high, generally starting at 25mg. In addition, the dose is often inconsistent when serum levels are measured. A compounding pharmacist will use micronized pregnenolone, usually made from plant products. The average dose I find effective in my practice is 10-25mg per day. I always use pregnenolone in combination with other natural hormones. Small doses of DHEA seem to improve the efficacy of pregnenolone.

Side Effects

I have observed very few side effects with the use of pregnenolone. A literature review failed to report any serious side effects from its use (in either animals or humans). The side effects I have observed are acne (very rare) and drowsiness. Both of these side effects are dose-related and ameliorated by lowering the dose.

Nutritional Support for the Adrenal Glands

Nutritional support for the adrenal glands is important to promote the production of pregnenolone. Dietary recommendations include: Vitamin C- 3000mg/day (one of the body's highest concentrations of Vitamin C is in the adrenal glands), Vitamin A- 5,000 I.U./day, Vitamin E- 400 I.U./day and Pantothenic Acid- 500mg/day.

[1] Sahelian, Ray. Pregnenolone, Nature's Feel Good Hormone. Avery Publishing. 1997

[2] Roberts, Eugene. Pregnenolone-From Selye to Alzheimer and a Model of the pregnenolone sulfate binding site on the GABA Receptor. Biochemical Pharmacology, Vol. 49, No. 1. P. 1-16, 1995

[3] Memory enhancing effects in male mice of pregnenolone and steroids metabolically derived from it. Proc. Natl. Acad. Sci. Mar. 1, 1992, 89 (5) p. 1567-71

[4] J.Steroid Biochm. Mol. Biol. Jul. 1994, 50(1-2), p91-100

[5] Sahelian, Ray. Pregnenolone, Nature's Feel Good Hormone. Avery Publishing. 1997

Chapter 13

Detoxification

This Chapter will explain why it is so important to detoxify our bodies—to rid ourselves of the various toxins we are exposed to on a daily basis. These toxins can result in hormonal imbalances that can lead to the development of chronic conditions including: arthritis, autoimmune disorders, cancer, chronic fatigue syndrome, fibromyalgia, etc.

I am certain that chronic illness and poor health is caused, in part, by the exposure to toxic elements that poison the cells of the immune system, the hormonal system, the nervous system, the cardiovascular system, and in fact, the whole body. A proper detoxification program can allow the body to get rid of the toxins and begin to heal itself.

One of the main organs affected by the exposure to toxic elements is the liver. The liver's job is to render these toxic agents harmless so that they can be excreted in the stool and the urine.

Problems develop when our detoxification pathways become overwhelmed as a result of overexposure to harmful chemicals. If the liver is unable to render these agents harmless, toxicity will build up in the liver and then move throughout the rest of the body. As the toxicity builds, more cellular damage occurs until the immune system is unable to do its job. This sets the stage for chronic illness to take hold.

It is vitally important to keep the detoxification pathways open and functioning optimally. The way to do this is to periodically use a proper detoxification program.

This chapter will detail the five steps of a detoxification program. They are:

1. Drinking adequate amounts of water
2. Heavy metal detoxification
3. Improving the diet
4. Sweating
5. Flushing the liver

1. Drinking Adequate Amounts of Water

It is impossible to detoxify the body without adequately hydrating the body. Water helps flush out toxins throughout the body, including the liver and the kidneys. Water also has healing properties of its own as it is able to carry nutrients into the cells.

It is best to drink most of the water between meals rather than at meals. To calculate how much water you should ingest, see Figure 11 on the next page.

Non-water beverages, including coffee, tea, and soda, can dehydrate the body. These beverages are not substitutes for water.

Drinking pure water, free of harmful chemicals such as fluoride, chlorine, pesticides, etc., is a must. I suggest using a water filter that removes all harmful chemicals and having your water checked periodically to ensure that the filter is functioning appropriately.

Fluoride

In many municipalities, fluoride is added to the water supply to help prevent cavities. However, fluoride is a known

Figure 11: Recommended Water Intake

1. Weight in pounds_____/2.
2. Result is recommended water intake in ounces.
3. Number of ounces _____/8 = _____ glasses of
    water per day.

carcinogen, and the dose of fluoride necessary to prevent cavities has never been accurately determined. In fact, studies consistently show little or no benefit from adding fluoride to the water supply.[1] [2] [3] Hardy Limeback, head of preventive dentistry at the University of Toronto, used to be an advocate for fluoridation. He now states, "Since April, 1999, I have publicly decried the addition of fluoride to drinking water." He feels there is no evidence of a benefit to fluoridation of the water and the long-term ingestion of fluoride may cause potential serious harm.[4] Dr. Limeback is correct. Fluoridation can cause harm.

An article in Medical Hypothesis found the amount of fluoride commonly added to the water supply can damage immune system cells.[5] Dr. John Yiamouyiannis, one of the world's foremost authorities on the effects of fluoridation, states that fluoride, in the amount added to drinking water, "inhibits over 100 different enzymes in the cells of people living in fluoridated areas." His research (with the chief chemist at the National Cancer Institute) estimated that fluoride added to the nations' water supply was responsible for 10,000 additional deaths from cancer per year.[6]   A recent study in the journal Brain Research showed that low doses of fluoride caused neurologic damage in rats.[7]

Fluoride and chlorine have also been shown to interfere with normal thyroid function by inhibiting iodine uptake in the thyroid gland.   Since many of the endocrine glands (e.g., the ovaries) normally have high concentrations of iodine, these agents may cause disruptions in the endocrine system. I have no doubt that the fluoridation of the water supply has dramatically increased the incidence of thyroid problems and other hormonal problems.

2. Heavy Metal Detoxification

Heavy metals can wreak havoc with the hormonal and immune systems. Heavy metals include:

A. Mercury

B. Lead

C. Cadmium

D. Arsenic

E. Nickel

I have found that a tremendous number of people suffering from chronic disease also have toxicity from heavy metals. Unless appropriate detoxification strategies are employed, the liver and other organs of the body will be functioning at a sub-optimal rate.

The U.S. Department of Health and Human Services lists

mercury as the third most toxic element known to mankind.[8] Because mercury is such a toxic element, all exposure to mercury should be minimized.

Dental amalgams (fillings) are the leading source of mercury toxicity. Amalgams contain approximately 50% mercury by weight. Other sources of mercury include immunizations (including the flu vaccine), fish, some pesticides and fungicides.

Mercury is a cell toxin that can disrupt the functioning of the entire hormonal system. The thyroid, hypothalamus and pituitary glands are very sensitive to mercury.

I do not recommend that fillings containing mercury be used for any reason. I recommend that you take extreme care in their removal. If you have mercury fillings already in place, only dentists trained in proper detoxification techniques should remove mercury fillings. Also, your physician can work with you to ensure that mercury levels will not climb as the fillings are removed. Removing mercury fillings without taking the proper precautions can cause an elevated mercury release in the body and immune system malfunction.

Mercury and other heavy metal detoxification requires extreme care and close monitoring. Monitoring should include measurement of pre- and post- levels of heavy metals to check progress. I prefer using urine challenge tests, including the use of DMSA, DMPS, and Glutathione. Supplements helpful in the detoxification process include: cilantro, Vitamin C, selenium, garlic and others.

3. Improving The Diet

Eating a clean diet, free of pesticides and hormones, is a must for a detoxification program. I encourage my patients to eat whole foods, with adequate amounts of protein. Eliminating the "whites"-- refined sugar, refined flour, and refined salt-- will help any health condition and help any detoxification program.

The glycemic index of carbohydrates can be a helpful guide on which carbohydrates to eat and which to avoid. The glycemic index measures how quickly carbohydrates are turned into sugar. Complex carbohydrates cause a much slower rise in blood sugar as compared to refined carbohydrates and are therefore a much healthier part of the diet. Complex carbohydrates have a very low glycemic index. Appendix A contains the glycemic index and can be used as a reference on which carbohydrates to eat.

In addition, it is vitally important to eliminate all refined oils in the diet. Refined oils contain trans fatty acids that poison our cell membranes and lead to degenerative disease. It is impossible to have properly functioning immune and hormonal systems while eating refined oils. Most supermarket oils are refined oils. Any oil sold in a clear container, without an expiration date, should be avoided.

Finally, I recommend eating only organic food. Organic food has more nutrients than conventionally prepared food. In addition, my own research has shown that organic food has fewer pesticides and heavy metals present.

4. Sweating

The ability to sweat is impaired in many individuals with chronic illness. Re-training the body to sweat is essential to stimulating the detoxification pathways of the body. I recommend using an infrared sauna to aid in this process.

Rubbing hydrogen peroxide on the skin, 10 minutes before a shower will stimulate the sweat glands and the lymph system. You can also add one cup of hydrogen peroxide to the bath water to help.

5. Flushing The Liver

A liver flush is a remarkable tool to help the body detoxify itself. Many times chronic illness will not improve until the liver is cleared of toxins. Some of my most difficult patients have not responded to any therapy until they have undergone a successful liver flush.

Flushing the liver of toxins can help improve the liver's ability to filter out harmful chemicals, activate and deactivate hormones, release and store glucose, increase the body's metabolism, improve digestion, and improve the functioning of the immune system.

Begin a liver flush by cleaning up the diet. As previously mentioned, this can be done by removing the "whites" in the diet (white sugar, flour, and salt). Substitute only whole foods and drink adequate amounts of filtered water. Having a massage therapist do a lymphatic drainage technique is also helpful.

The next step is to take butyric acid 500- 1,000mg three times per day and to use coconut butter, one tablespoon two times per day. These are healthy fats for the liver and are available at a health food store. Next, I recommend taking alpha lipoic acid 100mg twice per day. Adding in Vitamin C 5,000-10,000mg per day along with Taurine 500mg twice per day, will help. Finally, I have found that glutathione, given as an intravenous injection once per week, can rejuvenate the enzymes in the liver necessary for detoxification.

There are many items that are helpful for a liver flush. Listing them all is beyond the scope of this book. I caution the reader to work with a skilled health care practitioner when instituting a liver flush. You will get the best results when someone is there to guide you.

Final Thoughts

The idea of detoxification can seem daunting. Don't be overwhelmed. Find a knowledgeable health care provider who can work with you. A proper liver detoxification plan can reverse chronic illness and certainly will improve the functioning of the immune system and all the systems of the body. Two good books to read is _Detoxify or Die_ by Sherry Rogers, M.D. and The Detoxx Book by John Foster, M.D., Patricia Kane, PhD., and Neal Speight, M.D.

[1] Brunelle, J A, et al. Recent trends in dental caries in U.S. children and the effect of water fluoridation. J. Dent. Res. 1990 Feb;69 No. 723-7

[2] Gray, AS. Canadian Dental Association Journal. 1987. Oct:76-83

[3] Seppa, L, et al. Caries trends 1992-1998 in two low-fluoride Finnish towns formally with and without fluoridation. Caries Res. 2000, Nov-Dec;34(6):462-8

[4] Limeback, H. Why I am now officially opposed to adding fluoride to drinking water. April 2000. www.fluoridealert.org/limebasck.htm.

[5] Sutton, P.R.N. Is the ingestion of Fluoride an Immunosuppressive Practice? Medical Hypothesis, 1991, 35, 1-3

[6] Interview of Dr. Yiamouyiannis. Nutrition and Healing, Vol. 4, No. 11. November, 1997

[7] Verner, Julie, et al. Chronic administration of aluminum-fluoride or sodium-fluoride to rats in drinking water: alterations in neuronal and cerebrovascular integrity. Brain Research, Vol. 784:1998.

[8] ATSDR/EPA Priority List." Agency for Toxic Substances and Disease Registry. US Department of Health and Human Services, 1995

Chapter 14

Final Thoughts

When I wrote the first edition of *The Miracle of Natural Hormones,* I wrote the book to inform my patients and others of the successes that I have witnessed with the use of natural hormones. Now, five years later, I am more convinced than ever of their efficacy.

There is no reason to use conventional hormones when natural versions are readily available. The natural versions work better and do not cause the side effects seen with synthetic hormones. The Women's Health Study Initiative (Chapter 2) was the latest "nail in the coffin" for synthetic hormones. People are getting fed up with the side effects of synthetic drugs and are seeking natural alternatives. Natural hormones are one such alternative.

The proper balancing of the hormonal system has tremendous health benefits for everyone. This includes individuals with chronic illnesses as well as the people who are trying to age gracefully.

I believe that people do not have to suffer the ravages of illness or the toxicity of conventional treatments, nor do they have to be told there is nothing that can be done for them. The chronic conditions outlined in this book can be improved and, many times, cured through the use of natural hormones. Natural hormones can decrease the effects of aging and also enhance one's health and quality of life. Furthermore, natural hormones are extremely safe when used appropriately. Natural hormones in physiologic doses often have minimal or no side effects as compared to the toxicity of their synthetic counterparts.

I have chosen to present the natural hormones in this book individually, but I must stress the importance of using them in combination in order to achieve optimal results. The case studies I have included are all actual patients I have treated, and their responses to the natural hormones are genuine.

You might wonder why more physicians do not prescribe natural hormones. The answer to this question is fairly simple. In medical school, most physicians are never exposed to the uses and benefits of natural hormones or other natural treatments. Physicians receive most of their information on treatment options from studies funded by pharmaceutical companies. The research provided by these pharmaceutical companies contains no information on natural products. This is because natural items are not patentable products. In order for a substance to be patentable, it must be chemically altered. Pharmaceutical companies realize there is no huge profit potential in a natural product. They spend their time and money only on products that can be patented-- thus producing great profits. Therefore, little or no money is available for studies using natural hormones and other natural products. These same drug companies vigorously attack the studies that indicate the benefits of a natural product. Furthermore, no drug company will perform a study comparing a synthetic hormone to a natural hormone because the result would not typically be favorable to the synthetic hormone or the drug company.

I hope the case studies presented here can persuade both physicians and patients to consider the use of natural hormones to treat disease and promote health. The natural hormones should be used with the idea of promoting balance within the endocrine system.

The strongest argument I can make for the use of natural hormones is <u>THEY WORK</u>. They are safer and more effective than the synthetic versions. Every day in my practice, I see the positive results my patients receive from natural hormones. In addition, colleagues who also use these natural agents report similar positive results.

It is a common-sense argument that the body will respond more favorably to a natural hormone versus a synthetic hormone to treat disease and promote health. Dr. John Lee states it best, "It is extremely unlikely that man can synthesize a hormone better than the one nature derived from eons of natural selection."[1]

Natural hormones are already gaining ground in conventional medicine. In the future, I see natural hormones exerting a greater role in the practice of medicine in this country. They have to. The benefits of natural hormones and the lack of side effects are too compelling to ignore.

Lastly, I know of no better way to promote health and treat a variety of illnesses than through the use of natural hormones. The inevitable decline of hormone levels may be a signal for our bodies to begin the aging process. The proper supplementation of natural hormones along with a healthy lifestyle can reduce the negative effects of aging, improve the functioning of the immune system and effectively treat disease. The results that I see are genuine. They are positive outcomes taking place in real patients—people that are benefiting from a sensible, balanced and natural approach. As a physician, I am proud to be a part of this transformation.

To all of our health!

[1] Lee, John. IBID, 90

Appendix A: Glycemic Index of Carbohydrates

The glycemic index is a measure of the speed of entry of carbohydrates into the bloodstream. Since carbohydrates cause blood sugar to rise, resulting in an elevated insulin level, it is recommended to limit the foods with the highest glycemic index and to eat foods with the lowest glycemic index (i.e. those with an index <50%).

High glycemic index, greater than 100% ('Bad' carbohydrates)
Grain-Based Foods
> Puffed rice
> Corn flakes
> Puffed wheat
> Millet
> Instant rice
> Instant potato
> Microwave Potato
> French bread

Simple Sugars
> Maltose
> Glucose

Snacks
> Tofu ice cream
> Puffed-rice cakes

Glycemic Index Standard = 100%
> White Bread

Glycemic Index between 80 and 100%
Grain-based foods
> Grapenuts
> Whole wheat bread
> Rolled oats
> Oat bran
> Instant mashed potatoes

White rice
Brown rice
Muesli
Shredded wheat
Vegetables
Carrots
Parsnips
Corn
Fruits
Banana
Raisins
Apricots
Papaya
Mango
Snacks
Ice cream (low fat)
Corn chips
Rye crisps

Glycemic index between 50 and 80%

Grain-based foods
Spaghetti (white)
Spaghetti (whole wheat)
Pasta, other
Pumpernickel bread
All-bran cereal
Fruits
Orange
Orange juice
Vegetables
Peas
Pinto beans
Garbanzo beans
Kidney beans (canned)
Baked beans
Navy beans
Simple sugars
Lactose
Sucrose

Glycemic index between 30 and 50%

Grain based foods

Barley
Oatmeal (slow cooking)
Whole grain bread
Fruits
Apple
Apple juice
Applesauce
Pears
Grapes
Peaches
Vegetables
Kidney Beans (fresh)
Lentils
Black-eyed peas
Chick-peas
Lima beans
Tomato soup
Peas
Dairy Products
Ice cream (high fat)
Milk
Yogurt

Glycemic index less than 30% ('Good' carbohydrates)
Fruits
Cherries
Plums
Grapefruit
Simple sugars
Fructose
Vegetables
Soy beans
Nuts
Peanuts and other nuts

Recommended Reading List

The DHEA Breakthrough, by Stephen Cherniske, M.S.

Enter The Zone, by Barry Sears, Ph.D. (Harper-Collins, 1995).

Grow Young With HGH, by Ronald Katz, M.D. (Harper-Collins, 1997)

Hypothyroidism, The Unsuspected Illness, by Broda O. Barnes, M.D. (Harper and Row, 1976).

Living Well With Hypothyroidism, Mary J. Shomon (Avon Books, Inc. 2000)

Maximize Your Vitality and Potency, Jonathan Wright, M.D. and Lane Lenard, PhD (Smart Publications, 1999)

Melatonin: Nature's Sleeping Pill, by Ray Sahelian, M.D. (Avery, 1996).

Natural Hormone Replacement for Women over 45. Jonathan Wright, M.D. and John Morgenthaler. (Smart Publications, 1997)

Overcoming Arthritis, by David Brownstein, M.D. (Medical Alternatives Press, 2001)

Overcoming Thyroid Disorders, by David Brownstein, M.D. (Medical Alternatives Press, 2002)

Natural Progesterone. The Multiple Roles of a Remarkable Hormone, by John Lee, M.D. (BLL, 1993).

Safe Uses of Cortisol, by William Jeffries, M.D. (Thomas, 1996).

Solved: The Riddle of Illness, by Stephen Langer, M.D., and James F. Scheer. (Keats, 1995).

Testosterone Treatment of Cardiovascular Diseases. Principles and Clinical Experience, by Moller, J., and Einfeldt, H. (Springer-Verlag, 1994).

Other Resources

How To Find A Physician

For information on how to find a physician knowledgeable about using a holistic plan utilizing natural hormones, you can contact the following two organizations:

1. Broda O. Barnes, M.D. Research Foundation
   P.O. Box 98
   Trumbull, CT 06611
   (203) 261-2101
   www.brodabarnes.org

2. American College for the Advancement in Medicine
   23121 Verdugo Dr.
   Ste. 204
   Laguna Hills, CA 92653
   (800) 532-3688
   www.acam.org

How To Find A Compounding Pharmacist

Many natural hormones are available from a compounding pharmacist. To find a compounding pharmacist, contact the International Academy of Compounding Pharmacists at:

The International Academy of Compounding
Pharmacists (IACP)
P.O. Box 1365
Sugar Land, TX 77487
iacpinfo@iacprx.org
(800) 927-4227
Fax: 281-495-0602

Glossary

Adrenal glands: Either of a pair of endocrine organs located on top of the kidneys, which produce hormones, including DHEA and hydrocortisone.

Antioxidant: A substance that opposes oxidation reactions. These substances are believed to help reduce damage in the body caused by free radicals.

Circadian rhythm: Rhythm characterized by a 24-hour period or cycle.

Dehydroepiandrosterone (DHEA): An androgenic steroid primarily produced in the adrenal cortex. It is a precursor to other hormones including estrogen and testosterone. A Low level of DHEA in the blood may be a marker for many degenerative diseases.

Detoxification: The Process of removing toxins from the body.

Endocrine gland: A gland that produces an endocrine secretion commonly referred to as a hormone.

Endometriosis: The presence of functioning uterine tissue in places outside the uterus where it is not normally found.

Estradiol: One of three major forms of estrogen produced in the female body.

Estriol: One of three major forms of estrogen produced in the female body. It is primarily converted from estrone in the liver.

Estrogen: An entire group or class of steroid hormones produced primarily in the ovary; small amounts are also produced in the adrenal glands, testes and placenta. The three major forms of estrogen active in the female body are estrone, estradiol and estriol. Estrogen promotes the development of female secondary sex characteristics.

Estrone: One of three major forms of estrogen produced in the female body. It is converted from estradiol by biosynthesis, primarily by the adrenal glands.

Hormone: A product of living cells that circulates in the body fluids and produces a specific effect on the activity of cells remote from its point of origin.

Hot flash: A sudden sensation of heat caused by dilation of skin capillaries. Usually associated with an endocrine imbalance.

Human Growth Hormone: A hormone secreted episodically by the pituitary during the early hours of sleep, during exercise or in the case of injury.

Hyperthyroidism: Excessive production of thyroid hormone, resulting in an increased metabolic rate, tachycardia and high blood pressure.

Hypothalamus: A part of the brain that sits above the pituitary gland. It serves as the link between the nervous system and the hormonal or endocrine system.

Hypothyroidism: Inadequate production or utilization of thyroid hormone resulting in a myriad of symptoms including fatigue, a sense of coldness, atherosclerosis, menstrual irregularities, dry skin and others.

Hysterectomy: Surgical removal of the uterus.

IGF-1: A hormone secreted by the liver in direct response to growth hormone stimulation. It is commonly measured in the serum.

Jet Lag: A condition following long flights through several time zones and characterized by various psychological and physiological effects, such as fatigue and irritability. Jet lag can cause disruptions in the circadian rhythm.

LDL Cholesterol: Cholesterol bound to low-density lipoprotein. Often referred to as "bad" cholesterol because it transports cholesterol to the body tissues and increases the risk for heart disease, stroke and high blood pressure.

Luteal phase: The second half of the woman's menstrual cycle. During this phase, blood vessels and connective tissues in the lining of the uterus proliferate, readying the uterus for implantation of a fertilized egg. Progesterone is produced in increasing quantities during this part of the menstrual cycle.

Melatonin: A hormone produced by the pineal gland. It plays a role in regulating the body's circadian rhythm. Melatonin levels decline with aging. Melatonin is also a powerful antioxidant.

Menopause: The cessation of menstruation. Usually occurs between the ages of 46 and 55.

Night sweats: Profuse sweating during sleep that is a common symptom of the peri-menopausal state and is thought to be caused by a hormonal imbalance.

Osteoporosis: A condition characterized by a decrease in bone mass, resulting in porous and fragile bones. Hormonal imbalances and nutrient deficiencies are thought to lead to this condition.

Pharmacologic Doses: Refers to using doses of medications that exceed the body's own production of the particular substance. These high doses may make the body shut off its own production of the substance, resulting in the body becoming dependant on the exogenous source of that substance. Pharmacologic doses will lead to an increased chance of adverse side effects.

Physiologic Doses: Refers to doses of medications that do not exceed the body's own intrinsic production of the substance. Physiologic doses do not shut off the body's own production of the substance. The chances of negative side effects are much reduced when using physiologic versus pharmacologic doses.

Phytoestrogens: Compounds found in certain plants and which have estrogen-like properties.

Pineal gland: A gland located in the brain which produces melatonin and is thought to be a key factor in regulating the body's circadian rhythm. The gland is sensitive to light.

Pituitary: A small vascular endocrine organ located in the brain that regulates hormones which directly or indirectly effect most bodily functions.

Pregnenolone: A steroid hormone that is produced in the adrenal glands and in the brain. It is a precursor hormone to many of the adrenal hormones.

Progesterone: A hormone produced by the adrenal glands and the ovaries. It is integral to the menstrual cycle and pregnancy. Progesterone imbalances are often associated with premenstrual syndrome and osteoporosis.

Provera: A synthetic progesterone hormone.

Premarin: A synthetic conjugated estradiol hormone. It is made from the urine of pregnant mares.

Premenstrual syndrome (PMS): A syndrome often associated with too little of the hormone progesterone and a resulting imbalance between estrogen and progesterone. Symptoms include cramps, depression, emotional swings, painful breasts, food cravings, weight gain and bloating.

Recombinant DNA biotechnology: Technology in which specific DNA is inserted into bacteria where it is rapidly reproduced.

Steroids: Any of numerous compounds containing a 17-carbon 4-ring system, including a variety of hormones. They have a common structure based on the steroid nucleus.

Somatomedin-C: See IGF-1.

Testosterone: One of several anabolic, steroidal hormones produced by the adrenal cortex. When males reach puberty, the testes take over testosterone production and significantly increase its output. It has androgenic or masculinizing effects.

Transdermal cream: A cream that is applied and absorbed through the skin.

Index

E

endometrial cancer, 105, 109, 110, 111
endometriosis, 110, 111
estradiol, 105-108
estriol, 105-108
estrone, 105-108
estrogen, 93-94

F

fibroid tumors, 90-91,110, 122
fibromyalgia, 74.159-161
flouride, 51, 184-185
free radicals, 136

G

gangrene, 124
glycemic index, 188
goiter belt, 50-51
gotu kola, 154

H

human growth hormone, 155-170
hydrocortisone, 145-153
hypertension, 71-72,128, 129, 149, 152
hypothyroid,28-29,46-50

I

infertility, 35-37
iodine, 50-51
iron, 199

K

L

lead, 186
licorice root, 154

Serotonin, 133

T

testosterone, 110, 118, 120, 121, 122, 124, 125, 128, 129, 130,
trans fatty acids, 188
thyroid gland, 25, 40-41
thyroxine, 40-41
Triest, 106-107, 110
triiodothyronine, 41
Tryptophan, 133, 139-140

U

ulcerative colitis,70-71, 139

V

Vitamin A, 53, 79, 179
Vitamin B3, 53
Vitamin B6, 53
Vitamin C, 53, 79, 100, 112, 129, 136, 153, 179, 190
Vitamin D, 100, 112
Vitamin E, 53,79, 129, 153, 179

W

water, 184-186
Women's Health Initiative, 15-18

Books by David Brownstein, M.D.

More information: www.drbrownstein.com

The Statin Disaster

Statin drugs are the most profitable drugs in the history of Big Pharma. The best of the studies show statin drugs fail to significantly lower your risk of developing heart disease. This book will tell you the truth about statin drugs. Statins are associated with a host of adverse effects including:

- *ALS*
- *Breast Cancer*
- *Congestive Heart Failure*
- *Memory Loss*
- *Myopathy*
- *Neuropathy*
- *Sexual Dysfunction*
- *Skin Cancer*

Vitamin B12 for Health

Vitamin B12 deficiency is occurring in epidemic numbers. This book show you the many benefits of using natural, bioidentical forms of vitamin B12 and how B12 supplements can help you achieve your optimal health. B12 therapy can treat many common ailments including:

- Anemia
- Autoimmune Illness
- Blood Clots
- Brain Fog
- Cognitive Decline
- Depression
- Fatigue
- Fibromyalgia
- Heart Disease
- Muscle Disease
- Neurologic Problems
- Osteoporosis
- AND MUCH MORE!

IODINE: WHY YOU NEED IT, WHY YOU CAN'T LIVE WITHOUT IT, 5th EDITION

Iodine is the most misunderstood nutrient. Dr. Brownstein shows you the benefit of supplementing with iodine. Iodine deficiency is rampant. It is a world-wide problem and is at near epidemic levels in the United States. Most people wrongly assume that you get enough iodine from iodized salt. Dr. Brownstein convincingly shows you why it is vitally important to get your iodine levels measured. He shows you how iodine deficiency is related to:

- Breast cancer
- Hypothyroidism and Graves' disease
- Autoimmune illnesses
- Chronic Fatigue and Fibromyalgia
- Cancer of the prostate, ovaries, and much more!

OVERCOMING ARTHRITIS

Dr. Brownstein shows you how a holistic approach can help you overcome arthritis, fibromyalgia, chronic fatigue syndrome, and other conditions. This approach encompasses the use of:

- Allergy elimination
- Detoxification
- Diet
- Natural, bioidentical hormones
- Vitamins and minerals
- Water

DRUGS THAT DON'T WORK and NATURAL THERAPIES THAT DO, 2nd Edition

Dr. Brownstein's newest book will show you why the most commonly prescribed drugs may not be your best choice. Dr. Brownstein shows why drugs have so many adverse effects. The following conditions are covered in this book: high cholesterol levels, depression, GERD and reflux esophagitis, osteoporosis, inflammation, and hormone imbalances. He also gives examples of natural substances that can help the body heal.

See why the following drugs need to be avoided:

- Cholesterol-lowering drugs (statins such as Lipitor, Zocor, Mevacor, and Crestor and Zetia)
- Antidepressant drugs (SSRI's such as Prozac, Zoloft, Celexa, Paxil)
- Antacid drugs (H-2 blockers and PPI's such as Nexium, Prilosec, and Zantac)
- Osteoporosis drugs (Bisphosphonates such as Fosomax and Actonel, Zometa, and Boniva)
- Diabetes drugs (Metformin, Avandia, Glucotrol, etc.)
- Anti-inflammatory drugs (Celebrex, Vioxx, Motrin, Naprosyn, etc)
- Synthetic Hormones (Provera and Estrogen)

SALT YOUR WAY TO HEALTH , 2nd Edition

Dr. Brownstein dispels many of the myths of salt—salt is bad for you, salt causes hypertension. These are just a few of the myths Dr. Brownstein tackles in this book. He shows you how the right kind of salt--unrefined salt--can have a remarkable health benefit to the body. Refined salt is a toxic, devitalized substance for the body. Unrefined salt is a necessary ingredient for achieving your optimal health. See how adding unrefined salt to your diet can help you:

- Maintain a normal blood pressure
- Balance your hormones
- Optimize your immune system
- Lower your risk for heart disease
- Overcome chronic illness

THE MIRACLE OF NATURAL HORMONES, 3rd EDITION

Optimal health cannot be achieved with an imbalanced hormonal system. Dr. Brownstein's research on bioidentical hormones provides the reader with a plethora of information on the benefits of balancing the hormonal system with bioidentical, natural hormones. This book is in its third edition. This book gives actual case studies of the benefits of natural hormones.

See how balancing the hormonal system can help:

- Arthritis and autoimmune disorders
- Chronic fatigue syndrome and fibromyalgia
- Heart disease
- Hypothyroidism
- Menopausal symptoms
- And much more!

OVERCOMING THYROID DISORDERS, 3rd Edition

This book provides new insight into why thyroid disorders are frequently undiagnosed and how best to treat them. The holistic treatment plan outlined in this book will show you how safe and natural remedies can help improve your thyroid function and help you achieve your optimal health. NEW SECOND EDITION!

- Detoxification
- Diet
- Graves'
- Hashimoto's Disease
- Hypothyroidism
- And Much More!!

THE GUIDE TO HEALTHY EATING, 2nd Edition

Which food do you buy? Where to shop? How do you prepare food? This book will answer all of these questions and much more. Dr. Brownstein co-wrote this book with his nutritionist, Sheryl Shenefelt, C.N. Eating the healthiest way is the most important thing you can do. This book contains recipes and information on how best to feed your family. See how eating a healthier diet can help you:

- Avoid chronic illness
- Enhance your immune system
- Improve your family's nutrition

THE GUIDE TO A GLUTEN-FREE DIET, 2nd Edition

What would you say if 16% of the population (1/6) had a serious, life-threatening illness that was being diagnosed correctly only 3% of the time? Gluten-sensitivity is the most frequently missed diagnosis in the U.S. This book will show how you can incorporate a healthier lifestyle by becoming gluten-free.

- Why you should become gluten-free
- What illnesses are associated with gluten sensitivity
- How to shop and cook gluten-free

THE GUIDE TO A DAIRY-FREE DIET

This book will show you why dairy is not a healthy food. Dr. Brownstein and Sheryl Shenefelt, C.N., will provide you the information you need to become dairy free. This book will dispel the myth that dairy from pasteurized milk is a healthy food choice. In fact, it is a devitalized food source which needs to be avoided.

Read this book to see why common dairy foods including milk cause:

- **Osteoporosis**
- **Diabetes**
- **Allergies**
- **Asthma**
- **A Poor Immune System**

THE SOY DECEPTION

This book will dispel the myth that soy is a healthy food. Soy ingestion can cause a myriad of severe health issues. More information can be found online at: www.thesoydeception.com. Read this book to see why soy can cause:

- **Allergies**
- **Cancer**
- **Osteoporosis**
- **Thyroid Disorders**
- **A Poor Immune System**
- **And, Much More!**

The Skinny on Fats

The Skinny on Fats was written to educate you about the importance of consuming good sources of dietary fat. This book will teach you why we need fat and why we can't live without it. Good sources of dietary fat can:

- Prevent heart disease
- Promote weight loss
- Improve the immune system
- Help prevent chronic illness

Ozone: The Miracle Therapy

Ozone is one of the most powerful natural therapies that helps to oxygenate the body. Medical ozone therapy can be used to treat many common illnesses including:

- _Arthritis_
- _Cancer_
- _Infections_
- _And, much more!_